A Primer on
Dental Practice Management

Leslie E. Gaskins
The University of Florida
College of Dentistry

RESTON PUBLISHING COMPANY, INC.
A Prentice-Hall Company
Reston, Virginia

Library of Congress Cataloging in Publication Data

Gaskins, Leslie E.
  A primer on dental practice management.

  Includes index.
  1. Dentistry—Practice. I. Title. [DNLM:
1. Practice Management, Dental. WU 77 G248p]
RK58.G37   1985   617.6'0068   84-18062
ISBN 0-8359-5669-5

Production supervision/interior design: Tally Morgan

© 1985 by Reston Publishing Company, Inc.
A Prentice-Hall Company
Reston, Virginia 22090

All rights reserved. No part of this book may be
reproduced, in any way or by any means, without
permission in writing from the publisher.

10 9 8 7 6 5 4 3 2 1

Printed in the United States of America

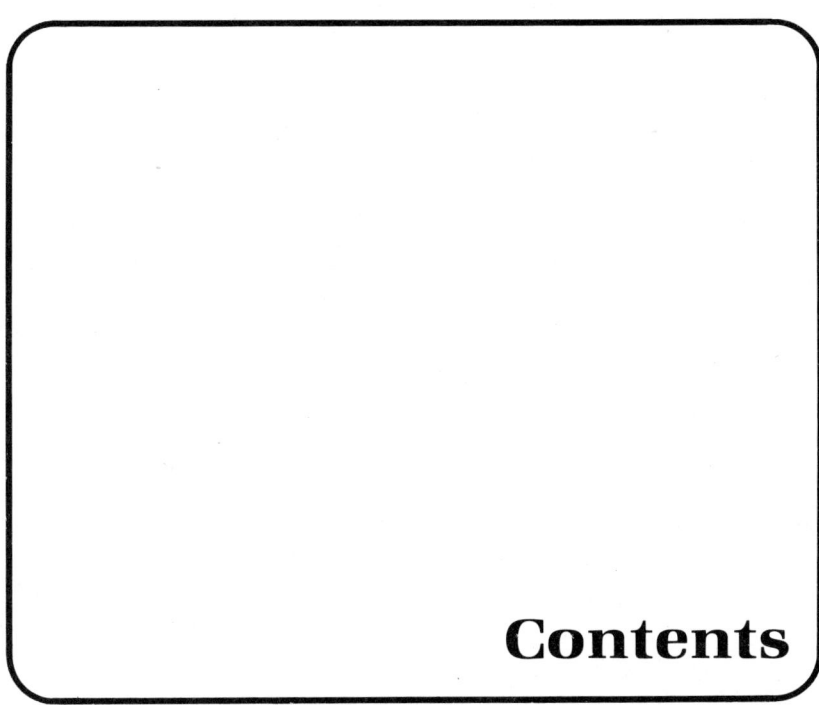

Preface, ix

1 PLANNING AND OBJECTIVE SETTING, 1

    Learning Objectives, 1
    Definition, 1
    The Planning Process, 3
    The MBO Cycle, 12
    Problem Solving and Innovative Objectives, 15
    Summary, 15
    Review Questions, 16

2 LOCATING YOUR PRACTICE, 17

    Learning Objectives, 17
    Factors Affecting Your Decision, 17
    Determining Location within the City or Area, 21

The Lease, 22
Summary, 24
Review Questions, 24

3 BUYING A PRACTICE, 25

Learning Objectives, 25
Advantages of Buying a Practice, 25
Disadvantages of Buying a Practice, 26
Evaluating a Practice for Purchase, 26
Pricing the Practice, 28
Negotiating the Purchase, 31
Summary, 32
Review Questions, 33

4 THE ASSOCIATESHIP, 35

Learning Objectives, 35
Advantages/Disadvantages, 35
Criteria for Success, 37
Contract Negotiations, 38
Summary, 47
Review Questions, 48

5 LEADERSHIP, 49

Learning Objectives, 49
Introduction, 49
Leadership Research, 50
The Hersey/Blanchard Theory of Leadership, 52
Definitions, 53
The Theory, 54
Theory Application, 56
Summary, 58
Review Questions, 59

6 COMMUNICATION IN A DENTAL PRACTICE, 61

Learning Objectives, 61
Introduction, 61
Ways of Communicating, 62
Staff Meetings, 64

Contents v

Summary, 70
Review Questions, 71

7 SMALL GROUP DYNAMICS, 71

Learning Objectives, 71
Introduction, 71
Group Characteristics, 72
Conflict Management, 76
Summary, 78
Review Questions, 78

8 STAFFING, 79

Learning Objectives, 79
Introduction, 79
Job Description, 80
Job Specifications, 81
Creating a Pool of Applicants, 82
The Selection Process, 82
Summary, 93
Review Questions, 93

9 DECISION MAKING, 95

Learning Objectives, 95
Introduction, 95
Vroom and Yetton's Decision-making Process, 96
Summary, 104
Review Questions, 104

10 PERFORMANCE APPRAISAL IN A DENTAL PRACTICE, 107

Learning Objectives, 107
Introduction, 107
Advantages of Performance Appraisal, 108
Dentist Personality and Performance Appraisal, 109
Motivational Aspects of Performance Appraisal, 111
Traditional vs. Effective Performance Appraisal, 112
Biases and Performance Appraisal, 113
Preparation for the Performance Appraisal Interview, 114
Common Errors in Performance Appraisal, 116

vi CONTENTS

Summary, 117
Review Questions, 117

11 MARKETING, 119

Learning Objectives, 119
Introduction, 119
The Marketing Plan, 120
Summary, 126
Review Questions, 127

12 PATIENT MANAGEMENT, 129

Learning Objectives, 129
The Purpose of Patient Management, 129
Philosophy of Patient Management, 130
The Appointment Plan, 132
The Appointment Book, 133
The Recall System, 134
The Problem Patient, 135
The Role of the Receptionist, 135
Summary, 136
Review Questions, 136

13 OFFICE RECORDKEEPING, 137

Learning Objectives, 137
The Office Recordkeeping System, 138
The Use of Credit, 145
Dental Insurance Programs, 150
Summary, 158
Review Questions, 159

14 FINANCIAL ANALYSIS, 161

Learning Objectives, 161
Introduction, 161
The Balance Sheet, 163
The Income Statement, 169
Ratio Analysis, 171
Cash Flow Budgeting, 174
Breakeven Analysis, 177

Summary, 183
Review Questions, 183

15 FEE SETTING, 185

Learning Objectives, 185
Introduction, 185
The Steps in Fee Setting, 187
Testing the Fee Using Breakeven Analysis, 190
Summary, 192
Review Questions, 192

16 INSURANCE, 193

Learning Objectives, 193
Introduction, 193
Protection of Earning Potential, 194
Types of Life Insurance, 196
Disability Insurance, 197
Medical Insurance, 198
Liability Insurance, 199
Summary, 201
Review Questions, 202

17 COMPUTERS IN A DENTAL PRACTICE, 203

Learning Objectives, 203
Introduction, 203
Computer System Options, 204
Microcomputer Components, 205
Determining Computer Requirements, 206
Procuring a Computer, 208
Summary, 209
Review Questions, 209

Index, 211

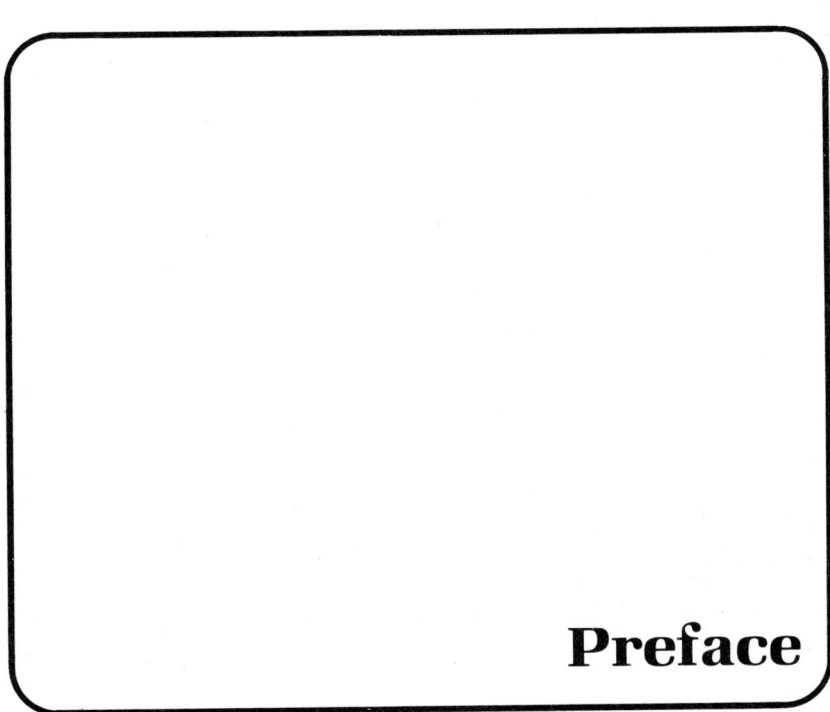

Preface

The purpose of this book is to serve as a source of information for dental students and dentists who either have had very little or no experience or who wish to review the basics of dental practice management.

The need for this book is well documented by the growing concern of practicing dentists over the increasing competition for patients. The last few years have seen a change from the past when almost any dentist could survive with little attention to management. Then, many dentists worked four or fewer days per week, at hours of their own choosing, and demanded cash for their services. Now dentists are being forced to extend their hours of availability to meet the desires of their patients and to accept the problems of extending credit. The ADA has emphasized the urgent need for training in practice management as have many of the other groups involved in dentistry.

Recently the Office of Health, Education and Welfare published a study titled *Private Practice Dental Delivery Systems* which may help to put practice management in perspective. The private practice dental delivery system is basically a self-supporting, entrepreneurial venture subject to financial investment risk and profit incentives. The practice must pay for itself to the degree that is congruent with the expectations of the owning dentist.

A dentist writing for the July 1981 edition of *Dental Economics* summed it up pretty well:

> Interpersonal relations, proper advertising, efficiency, quality dentistry, and how to make a profit are what we need in the 80's.

Within the space limitations of this book, we have to help you to practice successful dentistry, for if you do not, not only will you and your family suffer, but so will those who work for you, and most of all, you will have failed in your ethical responsibilities to your patients.

1
Planning and Objective Setting

Learning Objectives

Upon completion of this chapter, you should be able to:

- Describe the planning process.
- Explain how performance standards/goals are used in the control process.
- Discuss the motivational implications of goal setting.
- Describe the steps in implementing Management by Objectives in a dental practice.

Definition

In its simplest definition, planning means to decide in advance what must be done in the future. It is a means of bridging the gap from where you are now to where you want to go.

2 PLANNING AND OBJECTIVE SETTING

The importance of planning to the success of any business cannot be overemphasized. Management literature consistently stresses that the primary function of a manager is to guide the direction of his business by setting the goals and objectives to be attained, and, by forecasting the future to the best of his ability, to determine if the goals/objectives are feasible. He must then make the plans to achieve the goals/objectives and set up the controls which will tell him when the business is not following the plan or when the objectives are no longer appropriate. Finally, he must translate the goals and objectives into specific actions to be accomplished by the members of the organization.

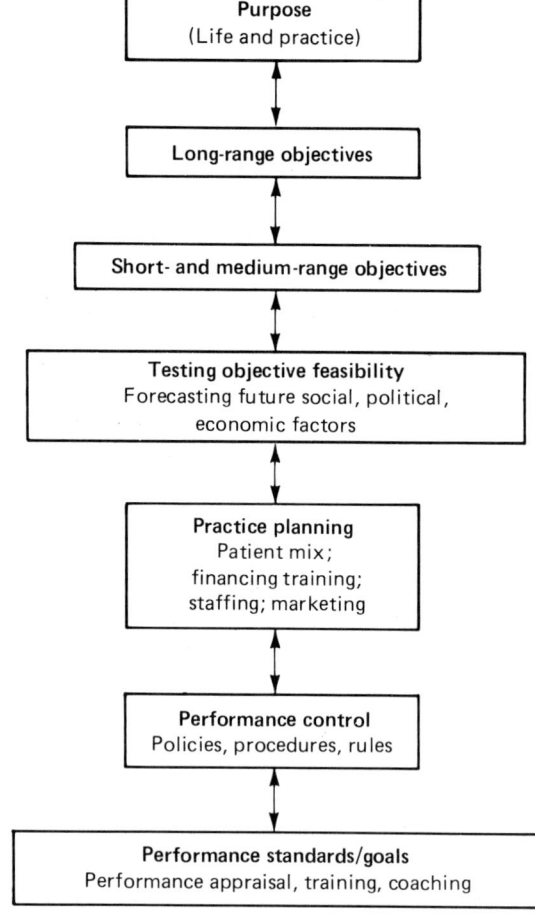

Figure 1-1 The planning process

Figure 1–1 depicts the planning process, performance standards/goals starting with the purpose and ending with staff development. It is important for you to note the use of the two-way arrows connecting each of the steps in the process to emphasize the interdependence of the steps. The process does not run straight from top to bottom, but rather runs in loops as you test each step to see that it supports the steps above it.

The Planning Process

Determining life and practice purpose

The planning process starts with a statement of purpose or reason for the existence of the practice. This should be derived from a statement of the purpose for your life. Although it is very important, because of time limitations we will deal only briefly with the broader issue of life planning and concentrate on business planning.

Figure 1–2 contains an example of a statement of life purpose. Your life's purpose reflects the values and goals you hold to be most important in your life. They may be difficult to define in writing, since many of us are not really conscious of our values and priorities. However, it is impor-

---
Life purpose

To be able to enjoy both my working and retirement years.

Goals
---

1. To be financially independent in 30 years.
2. To be a recognized authority in my field.
3. To provide effective and efficient dental care.

Forecast

Inflation will be 6 percent per year.
There will always be a market for my skills.
Dentistry will be increasingly subject to constraints.
   a. May become socialized
   b. Fees may be regulated
   c. Recurring licensing may be required
The population is aging — what impact will that have?
I will not become ill, disabled or die in the next 20 years.

Figure 1–2 Life planning

4 PLANNING AND OBJECTIVE SETTING

tant to your success and happiness that you define these values and the purpose for your life, for only if you understand your values and goals can you act consistently to attain them.

Notice how broad the life purpose statement is in Figure 1–2. It could mean different things to different people. Below the purpose are listed three possible goals which, if attained, might lead to the realization of the life purpose as *I* have interpreted it. Notice that the goals are still very broad, but not as broad as the statement of life purpose.

Now take a look at another set of goals derived from the same life purpose.

1. To earn enough money through the practice of dentistry to permit me to pursue my hobby of golf.
2. To become a championship professional golfer in 20 years.
3. To become the golf-teaching pro at the country club upon retirement from dentistry.

Figure 1–3 lists eight areas which should be considered in setting the goals necessary to achieve your life purpose. It is important to try to achieve a balance between these goals. You will not have enough time and resources to maximize goals in each of these eight areas. Increasing the emphasis on one goal can only be achieved by reducing the emphasis on one or more of the remaining goals. We have all read fiction and non-fiction accounts of the damage that can be done to your physical and mental well-being by overconcentration on one of these areas to the detriment of the others; Charles Dickens' Scrooge is perhaps one of the best-known examples.

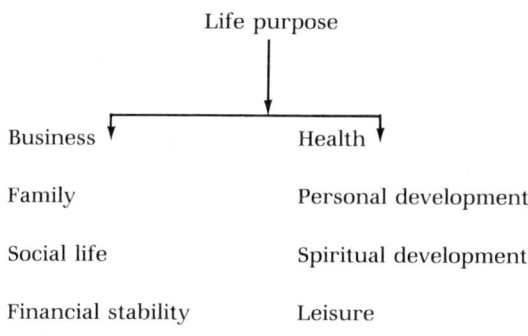

Figure 1–3 Areas for setting objectives

Setting practice objectives

Having discussed planning in its broadest sense, let us narrow the process to planning for your dental practice. As shown in Figure 1–1, the next two steps in the planning process are the setting of long-, medium-, and short-range objectives. Objectives serve as the means of organizing the remainder of the planning process. They are the ends toward which all activity in your practice should be aimed and which in turn support your life goals or practice goals. These objectives should serve as the basis for staffing, organizing, directing, and controlling your practice. Without objectives, your practice will lack yardsticks for evaluating practice performance and progress toward your goals. A 1981 American Dental Association (ADA) survey found that dentists who failed to set explicit objectives for themselves in the areas of practice management were unable to recognize problems because they lacked standards against which to judge the performance of their practice, themselves, and their staff.

The exact time period which differentiates between long-, medium-, and short-range objectives is not that important, but generally, short-range objectives are for one year or less. Medium-range objectives are for one year to five years, and long-range objectives are for any period more than five years.

The further into the future we try to look or forecast, the more uncertain we become about our assumptions of what is going to happen. Since we have evaluated the feasibility of our objectives based upon these assumptions, it is only logical that planning longer-range objectives entails more risk than planning short-range objectives.

As a general rule, the larger the organization, the less responsive to change it becomes. Since the large organizations are less responsive, the need for long-range planning becomes more critical. Companies like General Motors spend a great deal of effort in long-range planning. Because the dental practice is a relatively small business, it is normally flexible and responsive to change (if well managed). More time is spent in short- and medium-range planning than in long-range planning.

Management experts generally agree that there are eight objective areas common to all businesses.

- Marketing
- Innovation
- Human Organization
- Financial Resources
- Physical Resources

- Productivity
- Social Responsibility
- Profit

Marketing and innovation are the key objective areas; before all else, you must determine who your patients are, what their perceived needs are, and how you plan to meet those needs. As you will see in Chapter 2, "Locating Your Practice," you must decide what your product will be. That is, what type of practice do you want? A specialty? One that concentrates on crown and bridge? A preventive-oriented practice, or a purely general practice? You must make sure that the market for your type of practice exists in the locale that you have chosen.

The innovative objectives are closely related to the marketing objectives in that you must be innovative in finding new ways and techniques to attract and keep your patients. This requires that you keep abreast of technological and socio-psychological changes.

The next three objectives can generally be lumped together, at least in explanation. Human organization, financial, and physical resources must be obtained in order to meet the marketing and innovation objectives. The shopping for and attracting of the financial resources required to support your practice requires special skills, which will be discussed in Chapter 14. Unless you carefully plan for the physical layout of your practice, you will not be able to attract patients, nor treat them effectively. The decor must be attractive, and the principles of facility design must be adhered to. The human organization is equally important, for you must have objectives that will permit you to attract personnel with the necessary attitudes and skills to deliver effective dental care, or objectives that will enable you to develop the necessary skills and attitudes within your staff.

Having identified the areas in which we should set objectives, how exactly do we write the objectives? The writing of good objectives takes considerable thought and practice; however, adhering to the following criteria for good objectives will help. Effective objectives must be

- specific
- measurable
- comprehensive
- time-specific

Effective objectives must be specific and state exactly what is to be attained. "To make a profit" is not a good objective because it is not specific — it does not state the meaning of profit. Neither is the objective, "To make more money than I spend," for it does not say how much more money. "To make a profit of $10,000 by 1 January, 19XX" is an improvement over the first two objectives because it is specific in stating exactly what is to happen. It is measurable because we can count the number of dollars of profit we have on 1 January, 19XX, and it is time-specific.

The requirement that the objective be comprehensive is important because the attainment of a specific objective must not be done without regard for its impact upon other areas and objectives of the practice. Objectives must also specify what other conditions must be met outside the objective. For instance, an objective might be, "To gross $2,000 a month for the next twelve months." To make the objective comprehensive, we must qualify it as follows, "To gross $2,000 a month for the next twelve months without sacrificing quality or increasing stress."

Forecasting

Once you have determined the long-, medium-, and short-range objectives for your practice, you must now test the feasibility or attainability of those objectives. Many people feel that planning in an uncertain world is futile, and yet it is exactly because the world is so uncertain that planning is necessary. For unless you set objectives and test them for feasibility against your assumptions or your forecast of what the future will be like, you will be unable to cope with the unexpected.

For example, if you have a vague notion of retiring someday but have not set any objectives or done any planning for retirement, you are in a poor position to assess the effects of the unexpected — such as changes in the inflation rate and the current threats to Social Security. If you have set objectives and tested them against specific assumptions, you will find it easier to detect changes to those assumptions which could affect your plans. This process, formally called "forecasting," is the process of scanning the environment and making assumptions about conditions that will exist in the future that might affect attainment of your objectives.

Figure 1-4 presents a framework for outlining your assumptions, or making your forecast of the future. Here the dental practice is likened to a living organism that must cope successfully with its environment in order to survive. The practice takes in food or raw materials in the form of money (either borrowed or derived from services rendered), people in the form of patients, and staff personnel, equipment, and knowledge, to mention but a few of the inputs into the dental delivery system.

The dental practice processes the inputs and produces an output or product (oral health and patient satisfaction). If the product is acceptable

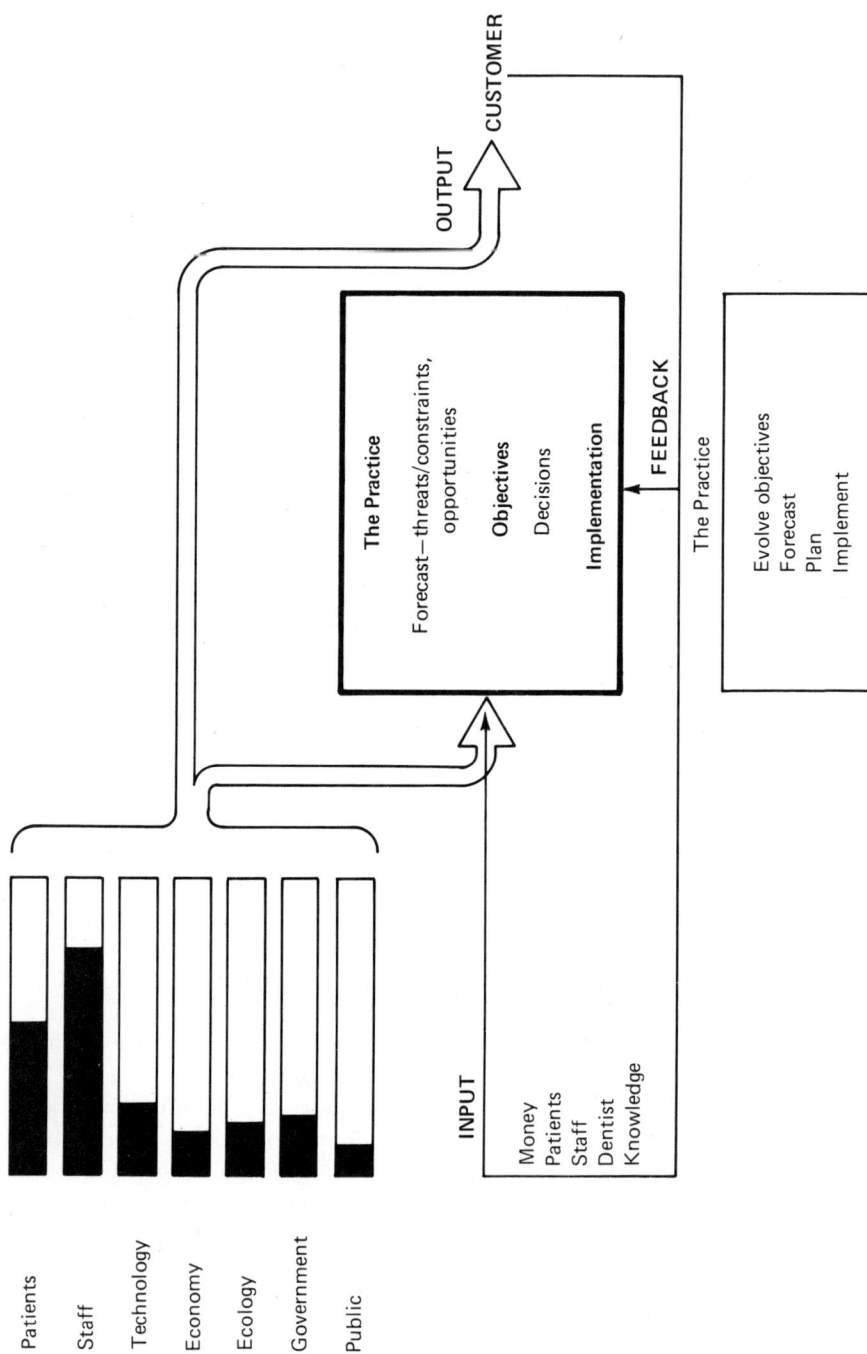

Figure 1-4 The dental system

to the market (the external environment), it generates new resources for the practice and the cycle repeats itself. Another input to the practice from the environment is feedback in the form of compliments, complaints, and data from marketing studies.

The cycle is not stable because it is affected by other elements in the environment. The upper left corner of Figure 1–4 lists some of those elements. The dark shaded portion of each of the bars in this part of the figure indicates an estimate of the amount of influence or control that you, the dentist, have over these elements. For example, you should have more influence over your staff than you do over your patients, and more influence over your patients than you do over the general public with whom you do not communicate. You may have influence over the government to the degree that you involve yourself in your dental society and politics. Political activity can have considerable impact on legislation affecting the practice of dentistry.

By listing as many of these environmental influences as you can think of, you can then make assumptions as to how they might affect attainment of your objectives. Figure 1–2 lists but a few of the assumptions as an example. By continually monitoring your assumptions and adjusting your objectives as the conditions change, you can vastly improve your probability of attaining your goals.

Planning action steps

The next step in Figure 1–1 is practice planning. This step entails developing the plans or action steps to assist you in attaining your objectives. For example, suppose that one of your short-range practice objectives was "To reduce the accounts receivable collection time to less than 60 days." (Accounts receivable is a term for the money owed you by your patients.) The plans, or actions required to achieve the objective, might be as follows:

1. To attempt to collect from each patient immediately upon the completion of the visit.
2. Where collection is not possible, to present a bill to the patient every 30 days until the full amount owed is collected.
3. To charge X% interest on all balances due more than 30 days to encourage early payment.
4. To make a series of follow-up telephone calls to patients with accounts overdue by more than 60 days.
5. To automatically issue a form letter to patients with accounts overdue by more than 180 days, warning that the account will be turned

over to a collection agency if no payment is received within two weeks.

We have set an objective that met all the specifications for an effective objective and then described the plan, or steps required to attain it. Now you must make certain assumptions about the future to insure that the objective is feasible, such as assuming:

1. That the skills and time available to your office staff will permit you to implement the steps.
2. That laws affecting the imposition of interest on loans will permit the charging of the amount of interest you stipulated.
3. That the steps you have outlined will not antagonize your patients and result in a loss of patients and decreased practice growth.

If any of these assumptions fail to hold, you will have to evaluate the possible impact of the change on probability and desirability of attaining your objective.

You have set the objectives which will guide the direction of your practice, tested the feasibility of reaching the objectives by forecasting the future environment to the best of your ability, and planned the actions required to attain those objectives. The next step in Figure 1-1 is that of performance control.

Performance control is the management function that enables you to compare the actual practice performance against desired progress toward reaching your practice objectives. This comparison can help you to discern and correct problems.

It is very seldom that all your assumptions will hold true and that the steps you have planned to achieve the objectives will work. When you discover these problems, two options are open: (1) to change or modify the objectives, or (2) to plan new action steps which will cope with the problems and put you back on course toward your objectives.

From the day you start your practice, you must have help from others to implement the plans and take the steps toward attaining your objectives. Once you have hired a staff, you have the problem of controlling their performance so that their efforts can assist you in attaining your practice goals.

Goal setting

"Setting performance standards and goals" is really a subpart of performance control, but because of its importance to the success of your practice, we have addressed it as a separate step. Once you have determined your practice objectives, you are faced with the problem of how to control and direct the efforts of your staff to assist you in attaining those objectives.

To provide effective control over worker performance, you need to be aware of the research on goal setting and how this research applies to your dental office. Research indicates that workers most often do not know what is expected of them and that this lack of knowledge is the major source of stress, dissatisfaction, and inefficiency.

The success of goal setting in controlling and improving worker performance is one of the most consistent findings in the management research literature. When your staff knows exactly what you want them to do and how well you want them to do it, their performance improves markedly.

However, these findings have led some management experts to draw unwarranted conclusions. For example, some conclude that worker participation in goal setting improves performance and that the goals set for the workers must be attainable to keep the worker from becoming frustrated and de-motivated. Actually, the evidence indicates that participation in setting the goals themselves does not improve performance, except when that participation results in setting a higher goal than you would have set without the worker's participation. (It is true that permitting the worker to participate in planning the steps or methods to be followed in attaining the goals does improve performance in most cases.) Further, setting impossibly high goals does not de-motivate the workers and does improve performance if you do not punish them for failing to attain the goal and if you reward them for improvements in performance.

Rewards must be contingent upon performance, and a smile, a kind word or a pat on the back will do wonders in this respect, but remember that major improvement in performance is gained by tying significant monetary reward to performance improvement. No system that I know of will provide something for nothing.

It is also not enough to set specific, hard goals unilaterally. You must also set up a control system to provide feedback, or knowledge of results required by your staff in order for them to correct their performance and so that you can reward them when performance improves. The research also indicates that feedback generated by the workers in evaluating their own performance against the goals is far more motivating than feedback that they receive from you as their superior.

Because of these research findings, you can see that control of worker performance is a natural outgrowth or extension of planning and objective setting. The use of objectives in the management of a business is called Management by Objectives (MBO), a technique used by an increasingly large number of businesses. The main thrust of management by objectives is to insure not only that the workers know what is expected of them in the form of performance objectives or performance standards, but also that they receive feedback on how well they are accomplishing the objectives, and that each of the workers' performance objectives aids in attaining the practice objectives.

The MBO Cycle

Define practice objectives

Figure 1-5 outlines the management by objective cycle. Starting in the upper left corner of the figure, you start the cycle by defining your practice objectives using the techniques discussed previously.

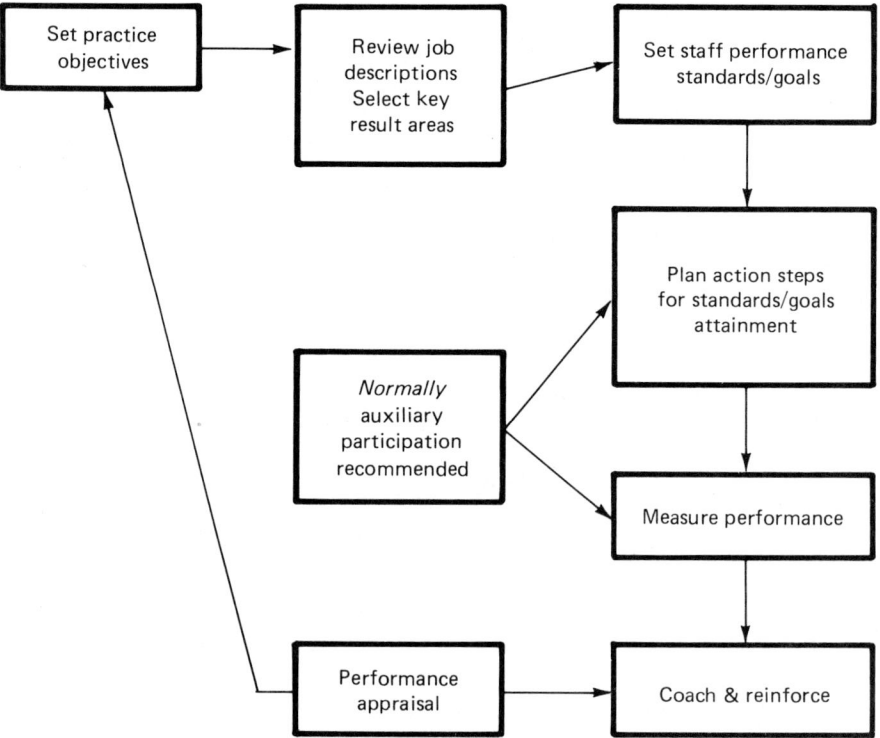

Figure 1-5 Management by objective process

Select key result areas

The next step is to review the job descriptions of the auxiliaries to select the key areas in which to set the auxiliary performance objectives. You must identify the key areas in order to place emphasis, or concentrate on the most important areas of the practice.

The reason for concentrating on a few key result areas rather than all the areas included in the job description is explained by the Pareto Principle. This principle states that 80 percent of the products in a business will produce only 20 percent of the profits. The reverse is also true: 20 percent of the products produce 80 percent of the profits. Similarly, 20 percent of the patients will make 80 percent of the complaints.

Keeping this rule in mind will help you to realize the importance of concentrating on those few key activities which will produce 80 percent of the progress toward your objectives.

By choosing only the key areas for emphasis, you will be able to see that they receive the priority attention they deserve from both you and your staff.

Set performance standards and goals

Once you have designated the key result areas, you must set the standards of performance and goals in those areas. Performance standards should describe the minimum performance you are willing to pay for. In other words, unless these standards can be met or exceeded, the auxiliary will be terminated. Some examples of performance standards are: (1) To take full mouth radiographs in 20 minutes with no more than a 10 percent rejection rate, or (2) Patient treatment will not be interrupted for the lack of complete armamentarium more than once in any two-week period. The goals, as contrasted to performance standards, should be the ideal performance that you want your auxiliaries to strive to attain in each key result area. Note that a time is not specified for the performance standards as it is for objectives. Time is used as one of the objective criteria only when a change is desired, i.e., when performance is to be improved, or a condition is to be attained. Performance standards do not require a time specification because they are minimum standards to be maintained or exceeded on a continuous basis.

Plan for goal attainment

While auxiliary participation in setting performance standards and goals is not necessary, auxiliary participation in planning the action steps for attaining the performance standards/goals has been found to improve per-

14   PLANNING AND OBJECTIVE SETTING

formance for two reasons. First, it insures auxiliary understanding of the performance standards/goals and the actions necessary to attain them. Second, it makes use of the auxiliary's job knowledge and expertise in planning for the performance standard/goal attainment. The auxiliary will often have a better understanding than you of the detailed problems to be encountered in performance standard/goal attainment.

Notice in Figure 1 5 that there are two areas in the management by objective cycle in which participation by the subordinate is normally recommended. It is important to emphasize the phrase *normally recommended*. A large amount of the literature on management by objectives assumes that subordinate participation in these areas will increase commitment, motivation, and performance. In the majority of the cases, this assumption will be true. However, research has shown that requiring participation in the MBO cycle can be threatening and de-motivating to workers who have low self-esteem, are authoritarians, or whose past experience has caused them to mistrust management. Auxiliary participation should be encouraged in planning for goal attainment and in measuring performance against the performance standards/goals, but you should not force reluctant employees to participate. It is recommended that performance standards/goals be set for all workers regardless of whether or not they participate in the planning and performance-measuring process. The least you can do is to insure that each auxiliary knows exactly what is expected of him or her and how that performance will be measured.

Measure performance

Setting of the performance standards and goals will be useless unless you set up an effective system for measuring the auxiliary's performance against the standards and goals. Such a system must be both accurate and simple. The auxiliary should be held responsible for recording the performance data and comparing it against the performance standards/goals since this will provide her with automatic feedback. As discussed, this should improve her performance more than if the feedback were received from you.

Coaching and reinforcement

In the process of measuring progress against the standards, you must provide the auxiliary with the necessary reinforcement and coaching to reach or exceed the performance standards and to get as close as possible to the performance goals.

Problem Solving and Innovative Objectives

In addition to the performance standards/goals which refer to the more routine operations of your practice, there are some other types of goals or objectives that will be necessary.

Problem-solving objectives are impermanent in nature and are implemented to cope with specific problems. Once the problem is solved, the objective is deleted or becomes a performance standard/goal.

For example, if the no-show rate is unacceptably high, an objective might be set "to reduce the no-show rate to 5 percent in 30 days." Actions to support this objective might be "to confirm 90 percent of the appointments the day before the appointment," and "to prepare a handout outlining the importance of keeping appointments, to be distributed to the patients within 30 days." If the objectives are met and the no-show rate is reduced, the objective might be deleted except for a performance standard requiring the receptionist to confirm all appointments 24 hours in advance.

Innovative objectives are objectives designed to improve the practice, such as "to conduct an attitude survey of all patients in the next 60 days for the purpose of identifying practice deficiencies."

An excellent description of the use of management by objectives in a dental practice appeared in an article by O. Marcotte, D.D.S., in the May 1980 edition of *Dental Economics*. He described his system as well-defined with everything in writing so that everyone on staff knows what they are doing, what results they expect, and how to measure those results. Their primary goals were: (1) "To help our patients keep their teeth for a lifetime;" (2) "Do the highest quality dentistry at a fair rate;" and (3) "To create an office environment where we feel proud to be professionals."

Dr. Marcotte's goals revolved around production collections, capital expenditures, and maintenance expense. At the end of 1979, he split the increased production profits equally among his staff.

Summary

The importance of planning in your function as a dentist/manager cannot be overemphasized. The planning process commences with the setting of goals for both your life and your practice. These goals provide the direction around which you plan the use of your resources. To be effective, your goals/objectives must be specific, measurable, comprehensive, and time-specific. Once the goals/objectives are set, they must be tested for feasibility against your forecast of future conditions which may affect their attainment. If your goals survive the test of feasibility, you must then plan the action steps to their attainment.

Management by objective, in the sense used here, is designed to control the performance of the practice and your staff to attain practice objectives. The steps in the process are:

1. Define practice objectives.
2. Identify key result areas in auxiliary job descriptions.
3. Set auxiliary performance standards/goals.
4. Plan the actions for attainment of performance standards/goals.
5. Measure performance and compare against performance standards/goals.
6. Coach and reinforce auxiliary personnel as necessary.
7. Conduct a formal, periodic performance appraisal interview with each staff member.

Goal setting is an effective means of controlling and improving auxiliary performance if it is applied correctly, based upon research findings.

Review Questions

1. Explain how planning can cope with uncertainty.
2. Explain how objectives or goals are used in the control process.
3. List and define the criteria for effective objectives.
4. Explain the difference between a performance standard and a goal when used to control auxiliary performance.
5. Describe the types of objectives and how they are used in a dental practice.

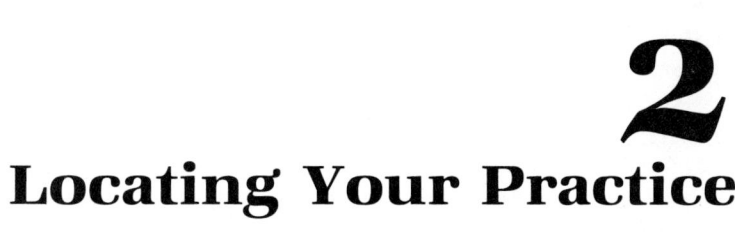

Locating Your Practice

Learning Objectives

Upon completion of this chapter, you should be able to:

- Discuss the factors to be considered in determining the market for dental care in a given location.
- Discuss the factors to be considered when choosing a location within a given locale or city.

Factors Affecting Your Decision

Locating your practice is one of your most important decisions. The seriousness of your decision is highlighted by recent estimates that changing the location of a dental practice entails an absolute minimum cost of about $25,000. The actual choice of a location will be based upon a mix of personal aspirations plus economic and professional considerations. This decision is now being further complicated by the advent of two-career marriages.

Personal factors

Considering your personal aspirations, some of the things that you need to think about are the achievements that you intend to accomplish during your career, i.e., what type of practice you would like — a large, high volume group practice or a small, rural practice. Do you enjoy a high pressure practice, or would you prefer a more relaxed pace?

Life style is another very important consideration. Everyone has a preference for certain types of climate, culture, and recreation. Some will prefer a rural life style and others, a suburban one. A large number of dentists make their home town their choice for location, and as we shall see, there is quite a bit of merit to this decision.

Economic factors

Once you've decided from the standpoint of your personal aspirations and preferences what kind of location you would like to have, and perhaps located such a place, major considerations still remain. Economic factors will affect the success or failure of your practice. Some of the items that you should be considering very seriously follow.

The basis for the economy in the area What is the source of income for most of the people in the area? Is it a single-industry based economy? If so, how stable do you think the demand for the industry's product will be? It is normally better to choose a location with a mixed economy showing economic growth.

An excellent illustration of the perils of a single-industry based economy occurred in the early 1960's at Cape Canaveral, Florida. The "Cape" had been enjoying a boom economy based upon the space program. However, the government decided to make drastic cuts in the space program, with the result that the newspapers were full of stories about highly paid engineers and other technicians who were forced to give up their high-paying jobs for low-paying jobs such as gas station attendant. From your standpoint, it should be obvious that if this sort of thing happens in your community, you will have a difficult time finding patients.

Disposable income Since most patients consider dental treatment to be a deferrable expense to be faced as a last resort, the demand for dental care will be highly dependent upon their disposable income. As disposable income decreases, one of the first items to be foregone is dental care. The extent of disposable income can be determined by checking on the amount of *demand deposits* available in the local banks.

Demand deposits is just another term for checking accounts. We assume that money in a checking account is money that individuals are willing to or plan to spend. This may change in the near future with the advent of the income-producing checking account. As the distinction between checking accounts becomes blurred, it will be harder to determine true disposable income. Another good indication of disposable income is the number of chain stores, restaurants and banks. These services have really accomplished your marketing survey for you, since disposable income, basis of economy, economic growth and so forth are the items considered by chain stores, restaurants and banks in determining the feasibility of new locations.

Economic and population growth trends These trends are very important items to check to insure that the economy is growing at least as fast as the inflation rate. Among the other economic factors to be considered are the cost of living and the tax structure, both for income and property taxes.

Demographic factors

Most of you have heard about the dentist-to-population ratio, which is available for broad locations, i.e. states, from the ADA publication "Distribution of Dentists in the United States by State, Region, and County." However, the dentist-to-population ratio is only one indicator of the demand for dental care. Beyond the dentist-to-population ratio you must be concerned with the socioeconomic factors that we have just mentioned, plus the demographics and dental IQ of the population. We have found that dental IQ varies proportionately with the education level and socioeconomic status.

To give you an example of the implications of the dentist-to-population ratio, you might consider that one-fifth of the population will normally never see a dentist. The average person will visit the dentist 1.5 times per year, and children under the age of 15 average three visits per person per year. However, from the ages of fifteen to forty-four, the average number of visits drops to .45 per year. In addition, non-Caucasians and the lower socioeconomic status members will only average .45 visits per year. It isn't just how many people there are per dentist that counts, it's the composition of the population. If you are interested in pedodontics or in a fixed and removable practice, you would want to look at the population from the standpoint of age.

Let us, for the moment, walk through a computation which would give us an idea of what the ideal dentist-to-population ratio would be, based upon the data that I have just given you. The average patient visits the dentist 1.5 times per year. The latest American Dental Association (ADA) survey indicates that the average dentist has 72 patient visits per week. Assuming we work 50 weeks out of the year with two weeks for a vacation, we would have 50 weeks times 72 patients, or 3,600 patient visits in a year. These 3,600 visits would require 3,600 divided by 1.5, or 2,400 patients. Considering that 10% of our available population will never visit the dentist, and 14% will visit only once in five years, we must conclude that 24% of our patient pool will not be active patients. Therefore, if we divide the 2,400 patient estimate by 76 percent, we will find that a pool of 3,157 patients is required to support the average 72 patient visits per week. It is interesting to note that in Florida, for example, the dentist-to-population ratio is 1 to 2,500. As the number of carious lesions in the population decreases, either the number of patients in the ratio must increase or you must provide other types of dental services, for example, periodontic or cosmetic dentistry.

Professional factors

The professional factors to be considered are your desired practice format and your compatibility with the population. You will probably have a preference as to the type of patient from both a cultural and demographic viewpoint because of its effect on your type of practice. Some dentists will only be comfortable treating members of their own socioeconomic class and will be unhappy treating patients whose class is either too far above or below their own, for each socioeconomic class has its own norms and cultural peculiarities. Some dentists will enjoy treating the full spectrum of patients from the very young to the very old, while others will feel a special affinity for a particular age group.

Prior to making a decision as to your practice location, you should do a marketing study to determine if the demographics and economic class of the population in the area meet your desires. Of course, the type of practice must be compatible with your location. You are not likely to be successful if you locate your pedodontic practice in a retirement community.

You must also consider the availability of staff, suppliers, and laboratories, and of facilities suitable for your practice. Some dentists have been unable to locate in the area of their first choice because of lack of facilities. Other things to consider are the other dentists in the area and their outlook. Are they hostile and cliquish, or are they welcoming you with open arms? Remember that you will have to live and, to some degree, compete with these people. Along the same line, what is the image or prestige of the dentists within the community? What are the state laws and regulations governing the delivery of dental care? Are you comfortable with expanded duty assistants or not? What kind of licensing problems and reciprocities are available? If you intend to continue your education, then you must also consider the availability of continuing education.

Determining Location within the City or Area

Once you've considered all these items and have decided on a general location, you must decide on the particular area within the city, within the block and within the building.

Accessibility is one of the most critical considerations. How close will you be to your patient population? It is better to measure proximity to your patients in terms of time rather than miles. Speed of traffic flow varies widely, particularly in the metropolitan areas. In one area, traveling a few miles could require a considerable length of time, while in another, the time required might be insignificant.

You must also consider the forms of transportation available and the problem of parking for you, your staff and your patients, for this is an item of growing scarcity. Lack of parking facilities can seriously increase your cancellation and no-show rates, especially in bad weather.

In addition, you should determine which way the city is growing, since you will want to put yourself in the path of the growth so that the population will not move on and leave you.

Visibility is another important consideration. One of the ideal locations, from the standpoint of visibility, is a joint medical-dental complex which not only provides visibility, but makes for easy referrals and will normally require only minimum alterations of the facility to accommodate the practice.

A shopping center is also a good location because of the frequency with which the average population visits that area and the availability of parking. You must be careful in leasing space in the shopping center to insure that competing shopping areas are not being planned which will cause the shopkeepers to move to new areas, leaving you stranded. Also ascertain that the area will be kept attractive from the standpoint of housekeeping and maintenance. Home offices do not fulfill the public image of the modern dental office and should be avoided if at all possible.

There are a number of sources of information to aid in locating a practice that you should know about. The local chamber of commerce will provide you with brochures and information on the area of your choice. You should consider, however, that the purpose of the chamber of commerce is to foster business for the local area and its members are sometimes prone to emphasize the positive picture and downplay the negative information on their area.

The ADA publication, "Distribution of Dentists in the United States by Region and State" is a good source for starting your search for a location if you have no particular preference. Since it does not provide information on dentist distribution below state level, it is of little use in the final decision.

A better ADA publication is "Facts About States for the Dentist Seeking a Location." It also has the limitation of not providing data below the state level, but it provides basically the same information as the previously mentioned publication plus considerably more useful information such as:

- Percentage of growth of the population
- Average net income of dentists in private practice
- State individual income tax rates
- Cost of doing business
- Professional licensing information

Another valuable source is the State Statistical Abstract published by the state universities and available in most of your libraries. These sources will provide the answers to most of the questions that you will be asking, particularly from the standpoint of economics and dentist-to-patient ratio. Dental supply houses and laboratories are another excellent source of information. The local telephone book, which will provide the most up-to-date confirmation of the number of active practicing dentists in the area, is also recommended. You will seldom find complete agreement between the sources, but the telephone directory is usually the most current.

Another way to check on the demand for dental care is to make a few calls to dentists in the area requesting an appointment and see what the waiting time is.

The Lease

Assuming that you've located the exact area in which you wish to locate and have decided not to build at this time, negotiating the lease becomes one of the next important considerations. Below is an abbreviated checklist, which should help you in negotiating the lease. You should ask yourself the following questions.

Does the lease:

1. Accurately describe the space?
2. Specify rent and method of payment?
3. Clearly specify liability?
4. Specify services provided?
5. Specify responsibility for code compliance?
6. Specify what happens to fixed property after lease termination?
7. Specify rights of reasonable entry?
8. Specify conditions under which lease may be terminated?
9. Specify terms for lease renewal?
10. Specify subleasing arrangements?
11. State date of occupancy?

Does the lease specify the exact rent and the method of payment? It's quite normal to request an additional month's rent as a deposit. Does the lease clearly specify who is liable if someone is injured on the property? Does it specify the services that will be provided by the lessor in terms of janitorial and custodial services? Does it specify the responsibility for compliance with the local building codes?

What happens to *real property* after the lease termination? *Real property* is that property which is fastened to the main structure, and since some of your dental equipment meets this fixed property definition, it should be very clearly delineated that it remains the property of the dentist in the event that the lease is cancelled. Does the lease specify the rights of reasonable entry? This means that the landlord will be denied entry except under very specific conditions which will eliminate the possibility of your trying to treat patients while the local carpenters and plumbers are tearing apart your ceiling. Does the lease also specify the conditions under which it may be terminated? There are some leases that permit termination for any actions "deemed unseemly" by the lessor and do not specify in detail what "unseemly" means.

Does it specify the terms for lease renewal? It should at least specify that the lease will be renewable. You must expect, however, that there will be some sort of an escalation clause to take care of inflation. It should also specify subleasing arrangements and an "escape clause" should you decide that you want to move or you become ill or disabled and wish to sublease the property or be released from the agreement. The lease should also very clearly specify the date of occupancy and the date from which the rental fee will be computed.

It is absolutely essential that you hire the services of a lawyer before negotiating a lease. However, hiring others to help you does not completely eliminate the risk of doing business. The more you personally know about the business elements of your practice, the greater your chances for success.

Summary

There are four major factors which may affect your choice of a practice location.

1. Personal aspirations and life style preferences
2. Economic factors
3. Demographic factors
4. Professional factors

Aside from your personal aspirations and preferences, you must determine the local market for your practice. The ideal conditions would exist in a locale with a high, stable, per capita disposable income which is derived from varied sources with a high growth potential. These factors influence the ability to pay for dental care. In addition, you will need a population with a high dental IQ so that they realize the importance of and will seek dental care. This dental IQ correlates highly with socioeconomic level and education.

Having determined a locale, your next concern is to find a location with high visibility, easily accessible to a high population growth area and which has ample parking facilities.

If you decide to lease a facility, this chapter provides a checklist along with a strong recommendation that the lease be negotiated with the aid of a lawyer.

Review Questions

1. List three professional factors to be considered when locating a practice.
2. Explain why the dentist-to-population ratio by itself is not adequate to determine the demand for dental care.
3. Discuss the factors to be considered when choosing a practice location within a given city.
4. Describe the ideal location for locating a dental practice from the standpoint of economics and demand for dentistry.

3
Buying a Practice

Learning Objectives

Upon completion of this chapter, you should be able to:

- Discuss the advantages of purchasing a practice versus opening one.
- Identify the elements of value when purchasing a practice and be able to assess their value.
- Evaluate the suitability of a practice for purchase.

Advantages of Buying a Practice

It is usually better to buy an existing practice with its cash flow and patients rather than starting one from scratch. This trend will probably continue as long as the competition from the growing number of dentists and the price of dental equipment continues to increase. Among the present advantages of purchasing an existing practice are:

1. Obtaining dental and office equipment at a reduced price.
2. Bypassing the frustration and rush attendant with starting a practice from scratch, i.e., selecting and installing equipment, coordinating with contractors and suppliers, recruiting and training the staff, and building patient flow.
3. Providing instant patients and income (but not necessarily profit).
4. An existing practice has a record indicating the probability of having a successful practice. No records to indicate probability of success are available when starting from scratch.
5. It is generally cheaper in the long run to purchase an existing practice than to start a practice.

Disadvantages of Buying a Practice

The purchase of an existing practice is not without some disadvantages, such as:

1. No choice of equipment or office design.
2. Equipment is older and used.
3. Patients may not accept you.
4. Maintaining an existing practice normally requires a higher productivity level to break even. However, experience indicates that productivity does not drop more than 15 percent under a new dentist.
5. Fee schedules may be too low, or credit policies too lenient. Attempting to correct either condition as the new dentist may cause you to lose patients.

Evaluating a Practice for Purchase

There are a number of items that must be carefully examined to determine whether a practice is suitable for purchase. The first few items are the same as those involved in locating a practice. Does the location match your personal preferences, i.e., rural vs. urban, cultural activities, climate, recreational activities, educational facilities, cost of living index, and crime rate? Will the population and economic conditions continue to support a practice? What are the area economic trends and population growth rates?

Looking at the practice itself, what is the seller's reputation for business skills and reliability among other dentists, with suppliers, creditors, and the local banker? What is the quality of the dentistry performed? Can you examine some of the patients to determine the quality for yourself? Are the majority of the procedures accomplished in the existing practice procedures that you enjoy doing? What is the dental I.Q. of the patient pool as indicated by such items as their acceptance of crown and bridge and their response to the recall system? Are the patients the types of patients that you will enjoy treating — that is, are their backgrounds and values similar to yours?

Particularly in the older urban practices, look at the area where the patients live in relation to the practice location. The patients may have moved to the suburbs away from the practice location over the years and now make the trip to the same dentist only out of loyalty or habit. They may switch to another dentist closer to home if the old dentist is no longer available. Is your personality similar to that of the seller so that you will be compatible with the existing patients? Does the practice rely upon any contacts with special groups such as church or fraternal organizations, or upon your level of community involvement for its referrals and practice growth? If so, can you and are you willing to join those groups and continue a high level of involvement?

A step-by-step review of the procedures for handling new patients and a careful examination of the dental records will give you a much better feel for the quality of the practice.

For purely financial considerations, a healthy practice should have the following characteristics: The percent of collection should be between 95 and 98 percent. The amount tied up in accounts receivable will vary with economic conditions, tending to increase in recessions and decrease under normal conditions, but on the average should be between 12 and 17 percent of the gross income. The net income should be increasing at a rate at least equal to the annual inflation rate, and the fee schedule should be on a par with that of other dentists in the community. If the net income is not growing faster than inflation, it is advisable to examine the number of hours being worked. Many older dentists tend to decrease their operating hours so that while the practice has growth potential, income has been limited by the reduced hours. Also, if part of the problem is due to below average fees, consider what impact increasing fees will have on future practice growth and patient acceptance.

A CPA should be hired to review the condition of the internal bookkeeping. While you will seldom find a practice whose bookkeeping even approaches the ideal, the closer the practice approaches this ideal, the better its management. The ideal practice bookkeeping system should provide a clear and complete audit trail from the appointment book to the day sheet, to the bank account, and from the bank account to the disbursement journal to the expensing invoice.

For example, if Mrs. Murphy is shown in the appointment book on a given date, the day sheet should indicate what treatment was rendered to Mrs. Murphy, how much she was charged, and how and when she paid. Further, the amount she paid should appear on the daily bank deposit slip for that day.

All expenses except those from petty cash should have been paid by check from the disbursement journal, and the reason for the expense plus the invoice number recorded in that journal. At the same time, overhead and other operating ratios should be examined (as outlined in Chapter 14) to determine the efficiency of the practice.

Pricing the Practice

Once it has been decided that the practice meets your requirements, the next problem is to negotiate a fair price for the purchase of the practice. There are four or possibly five elements which together make up the fair market value: (1) equipment and supplies, (2) the restrictive covenant, (3) accounts receivable, (4) goodwill, and (5) leasehold improvements.

The fair market value of the equipment is best determined by obtaining an appraisal from a reputable dental supplier. In general, however, expect the equipment to be appraised at a higher value than the equipment could be sold for elsewhere. The increased cost is worth it since it will save the time and expense of shipping and installation.

There are some general guidelines to check against the appraisal. The normal lifetime of most dental equipment averages 20 years (10 years for tax purposes). It is estimated that the fair market value decreases to 40 percent of original value in five years and to 15–20 percent of value in 10 years, after which there is little or no further depreciation. For example, a $1,000 item of equipment will be worth approximately $400 at the end of five years, and between $150 and $200 at the end of 10 years, after which its value remains approximately the same for the remainder of its usable life.

Another item of value to be considered is the disposition of existing supplies, both office and dental. You should compare the asking prices with available prices in the supply catalogs. Be especially careful to consider the shelf life on perishable items such as anesthesia, and consider the quality of the brand items. Compare the amount to be sold with your expected consumption rate to be sure that you are not being overstocked and that you will have a use for the items. There is no joy in later discovering that you have 120 burrs of a type you never use.

The restrictive covenant is a promise by the seller not to set up a practice within a certain radius of the original practice for a specified period of years. The exact terms of the covenant and other implications will be discussed in Chapter 4.

It may be desirable to purchase the accounts receivable (A/R) at a discount to provide for increased cash flow. If so, the A/R should be aged, which is a process of evaluating the value of the A/R depending on the amount of time the A/R has been outstanding. The general practice is to sort the A/R into categories of 30, 60, 90, and over 90 days. Some experts recommend multiplying those under 90 days by the collection rate, which is usually between 90 and 100 percent. For those over 90 days, either do not purchase or offer 50 percent of value. Other consultants are more conservative and recommend applying the collection rate to the 30–60 day accounts and 50 percent to all accounts over 60 days. Still others recommend not buying the A/R at all because of the administrative expense and risk of incurring bad debts.

Another item which may contribute to the fair market value is leasehold improvements. Leasehold improvements are those physical changes that have been made in the facility to accommodate the dental practice. The best way to determine the value of these improvements is through an appraisal. In general, considering inflation, you can expect the present value of the leasehold improvements to exceed their original cost.

Goodwill covers all other considerations of monetary value other than the four just mentioned, i.e., transferability of patients, seller's willingness to assist in the transfer, source of referrals, location, quality of retained employees, fee schedules and collection ratios. In other words, goodwill is those items that make the practice attractive enough to the buyer that he will pay more for the practice than the sum of the previously mentioned tangible items.

There are a number of ways of putting all these factors together; for example, the following formula is suggested by Dr. J. E. Dunlap in *The Beginning Dental Practice*. To the fair market value of the equipment, supplies, and the leasehold improvements add last year's net income divided

30 BUYING A PRACTICE

by 10 plus last year's net divided by 20, and multiply by the number of months the seller is willing to stay with the practice after the sale in order to aid in the transition.

Consider the following example:

> Dr. Brown has been in practice five years and still owns his original equipment, which he purchased new for $25,000. His supply inventory totals $1,500, and you have decided that you need to purchase these supplies. Dr. Brown has grossed $57,000 in each of the last two years, with a 55 percent overhead. You have had a real estate appraiser evaluate the leasehold improvements at $10,000. Dr. Brown has agreed to remain with you for two months after the sale in order to help in the transition.
>
> To compute the value of the five-year-old equipment, multiply the original purchase price by 40 percent (.40 × $25,000) to obtain $10,000. To this add the value of supplies based upon an inventory of $1,500, plus the appraised value of the leasehold improvements.
>
> The net income is determined by subtracting the overhead (.55 × $57,000 = $31,350) from the gross ($57,000) to obtain the net income $25,650. We can now apply these figures to Dr. Dunlap's formula.

$$\text{Value of equipment and supplies}$$
$$+$$
$$\text{Value of leasehold improvements}$$
$$+$$
$$\frac{\text{Last year's net}}{10}$$
$$+$$
$$\frac{\text{Last year's net}}{20} \times \begin{array}{l}\text{months seller} \\ \text{will remain} \\ \text{with practice}\end{array}$$

Substituting we have:

$$\$10,000 + \$1,500 + \$10,000$$
$$+$$
$$\frac{\$25,650}{10}$$
$$+$$
$$\frac{\$25,650 \times 2}{20}$$

Consolidating the formula we have:

$$\$21,500$$
$$+$$
$$\$2,565$$
$$+$$
$$\$2,565$$

$$\text{TOTAL value of practice} = \$26,630$$

Still another method is to use two to three months' gross earnings plus the value of equipment, supplies, and leasehold improvements. Applying this formula, the same practice would be valued at between $31,000 and $35,750, which is considerably more than Dunlap's evaluation. However, remember that gross earnings alone are not a sufficient basis for determining practice worth.

Negotiating the Purchase

If the price can be agreed upon, the next step is the negotiation of the sales agreement, which should *never* be done without the aid of a lawyer and a consultant.

The agreement must specify the price for each category listed in the sale. If not, the IRS will make their own allocations of cost for tax purposes, which may not be at all to your advantage. For example, goodwill is not a depreciable item for the buyer but is capital gain for the seller. Therefore, the more of the price that is allocated to goodwill, the more advantage to the seller and the less advantage to the buyer. A way to handle goodwill which will benefit both the buyer and seller is to divide the number of dental records into the agreed upon value of goodwill to arrive at a cost per dental record. The buyer then pays for the dental records which are depreciable for tax purposes to the buyer and still remain as capital gains for the seller. Costs for equipment may be taken as an initial tax credit plus annual depreciation for the buyer. Also, the buyer may depreciate the cost of the restrictive covenant over the period the covenant remains in force. That is, if $5,000 were paid for a five-year restrictive covenant, the value may be depreciated by $1,000 each year for five years using the straight-line depreciation method. It is to the advantage of both the buyer and the seller to consider the tax implications of the sales contract. Because tax laws change so frequently, further discussion here is not warranted.

The following are also important points to consider in the agreement:

- The agreement can be made contingent on the buyer being able to obtain a loan within a specified time, after which the agreement is void.
- The agreement should require that the seller send an announcement of the sale to all patients of record and to all creditors of the practice to insure better transferability of patients and prevent the possible exercise of lien against the practice by creditors.
- There should be a provision to pay off the loan early without penalty should the buyer so decide. There should also be clear definitions of what constitutes a default of payment and what actions may be taken in the event of default.
- Responsibility for disposition of records must be made with the buyer agreeing to make reasonable access to the records available to the seller.
- Arrangements must be made for death or disability of the buyer, normally through an insurance policy in the amount of the unpaid balance.
- An agreement should be made specifying how complaints from patients treated by the seller are to be handled.
- If the A/Rs are not bought by the buyer, it should be determined if collections will be made by the buyer for a service fee, or if they will remain the sole responsibility of the seller.
- All the above should be contingent on the buyer being able to negotiate an acceptable lease agreement with the lessor if the property is not owned by the seller.

Summary

While there are both advantages and disadvantages to purchasing a practice versus starting a practice, in general it is better to purchase a practice. Your success will depend to a large degree on how carefully you evaluate the desirability of the practice — considering the reputation of the former owner, the type of patients, and the quality of both the dentistry and the practice management. It is equally important to negotiate a fair agreement for purchase, which should not be attempted without a good lawyer and careful consideration of the tax implications.

Review Questions

1. What are the items of value in a dental practice?
2. Discuss the various ways of negotiating for accounts receivable when purchasing a practice.
3. Given the following information, estimate the value of this practice.

   Dr. Jones has been in practice 10 years and still owns his original equipment, which he purchased new for $35,000. His supply inventory is evaluated at $1,000, and his leasehold improvements at $17,000. He has grossed $100,000 in each of the last two years, with an overhead of 60 percent and a collection ratio of 98%. Dr. Jones will not be available to introduce you to his former patients. In addition, you are interested in making Dr. Jones an offer for his accounts receivable which, upon being aged, are as follows: less than 30 days, $8,000; 30 to 60 days, $5,000; 60–90 days, $3,000; and over 90 days, $6,000.

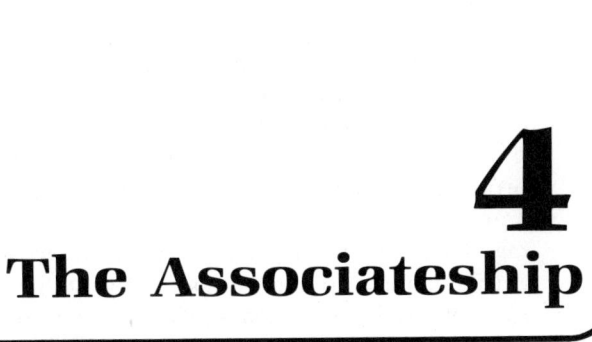

4

The Associateship

Learning Objectives

Upon completion of this chapter, you should be able to:

- Discuss the advantages and disadvantages of an associateship.
- Discuss the criteria for a successful associateship.
- Discuss the considerations involved in negotiating an associateship contract.
- Evaluate the financial implications of an associateship contract.

Advantages/Disadvantages

With the growing costs of setting up a practice, many dentists are turning to the associateship as a means of increasing productivity without a proportionate increase in overhead. This mode of practice offers a new dentist many advantages over the solo practice:

1. The young dentist is taken into a ready-made, ongoing practice and can take advantage of the patient flow created by the senior dentist. This results in instant cash flow with little risk and no capital investment. A recent study found that it required approximately four years for the dentist starting in a solo practice to equal the patient flow of a dentist starting in an associateship. In the meantime, the associate had started with a much higher patient flow and cash flow.

2. If properly managed, two dentists can increase productivity without a corresponding increase in overhead. Now, most dental facilities are underutilized, with approximately 40 hours of utilization per week out of a possible 168, or approximately 25 percent of capacity. Granted that there is little use for office hours between 11 PM and 5 AM, there are still many opportunities for increased productivity by making dentistry more available. The fixed overhead (rent, utilities, phone, insurance, etc.) may be likened to a "time cost" in that the costs continue to accumulate with time whether there is any productive activity or not. For example, if the fixed cost of operating a practice is $1,000 per week and the office is open 40 hours grossing $2,000, the ratio of fixed expense to gross income is 50 percent. If two dentists operate the office for 60 hours grossing $4,000, the ratio of fixed cost to gross income is now only 25 percent.

3. Additional economies may be realized by buying supplies in increased quantities to take advantage of reduced prices, and with the increased cash flow, it should be possible to obtain discounts for cash, or reduced interest for early payment of expenses. The sharing of personnel may also reduce costs through the sharing of receptionists, assistants, and hygienists.

4. In the less quantitative areas, it makes vacations and time for professional development more easily attainable, provides for free consultation, plus more flexibility in the office schedule through a sharing of emergency coverage and hours of operation. Perhaps even more importantly, it provides the camaraderie and the peer pressure to produce high quality dentistry.

Despite all its advantages, there are some serious pitfalls to the associateship:

1. An associate is, in fact, a synonym for employee. As it relates to dentistry, there may be a loss of individuality and freedom of action. The amount of restraint depends largely on the personality of the

senior dentist. The working arrangement can range from the senior dentist considering the associate as nothing more than a lackey or service apprentice to that of a peer relationship.
2. It is important to take time to become well-acquainted before entering an associateship. Too often the associateship terminates in personality clashes and bitterness for both parties.
3. The senior dentist must expect, and be able to cope with, the increased management problems that go with increasing the size of the practice.
4. The junior dentist must be prepared to accept a subordinate role in the practice, at least in the early stages of the associateship until he has gained the confidence of the senior dentist.

Criteria for Success

There are several criteria that must be met if the associateship is to be successful.

1. There must be professional compatibility with close agreement between the senior and junior member on the philosophy of practice.
2. There must be enough patient flow into the practice to provide an adequate income for both dentists.
3. The staff must be adequate in number and sufficiently trained to support the increased patient flow. It is also important to insure that the new dentist and the staff are psychologically compatible.
4. The facilities must be able to sustain the increased patient flow, with special attention to the size of the reception area.
5. The junior member must carefully evaluate his growth potential in the practice, and the senior dentist must be willing to share both patients and some degree of authority. Further, the mix of patients and procedures assigned to the associate must broaden his experience and assist in his technical development.
6. The senior dentist must be a good manager with neat and complete dental and financial records. The accounts receivable (A/R) collection rate should be greater than 96 percent, and no more than two months' gross production should be tied up in the A/R. At this writing, overhead should not exceed a maximum of 60–65 percent.

Contract Negotiations

The balance of this chapter discusses items which should be covered in the negotiations.

Will an assistant be furnished, and if so, who will pay for her, and who will she be responsible to (the senior or junior member)? It is normally better for the junior dentist to hire his own assistant and, if the senior dentist wishes to pay her salary, to do so indirectly by adjusting the junior dentist's compensation, for it will be difficult for the associate to assert his authority over an assistant when her pay and future are controlled by the senior dentist.

What will be the policy on assignment, acceptance and refusal of patients? Will the senior member assign a portion of the new patients to the junior member as they enter the patient pool, or will the senior member reserve the right to hand pick the patients to be assigned to the junior member, and will the junior member have the freedom to accept or reject these patients?

Will the after-hours and emergency coverage be shared, or will these duties all fall to the junior member?

Compensation

How will the junior member be paid? There are a number of arrangements and combinations for determining how the junior member will be paid. It may be a strict salary arrangement or some portion of production. It is almost impossible to cover all the possible combinations, or to say which one is best for the junior member. For example, the junior member could receive a flat 35 percent of either gross or collected production. Another arrangement could be 45 percent of gross or collected production less one half of the lab fees.

An important consideration is whether the percentage will be based upon gross or collected production. It is to the junior member's advantage to base income on gross production because his payment does not depend upon the ability of the office staff to collect from the patient. Basing the percent on collected gross may be to the senior dentist's advantage, since it prevents the junior member from providing dentistry to patients who cannot pay.

One of the best ways to determine an equitable percentage of production for the junior member is to work out some typical cases to see how both sides will fare under the arrangement.

NOTE: We recommend that you read Chapter 14 prior to reading the following section in order to better understand the concepts and terminology presented.

From your reading of Chapter 14, you will remember the breakeven formula:

$$\text{Breakeven} = \frac{\text{fixed expense} + \text{desired net income}}{(1 - \text{variable expense ratio})}$$

To illustrate the use of this formula in evaluating the financial aspects of the associateship agreement, let us take a typical example.

An established dentist, whose financial situation is as depicted in Figures 4–1 and 4–2, has decided to enter into an associateship agreement with another dentist. By the terms of the proposed agreement, the senior dentist has agreed to hire and pay $10,000 per year for another dental assistant to support the new associate. In addition, he agrees to pay the new associate 40 percent of his collected gross. Assume that the new associate will be an independent contractor so that the senior dentist will not have to pay for social security, unemployment compensation, nor have to include him in any of the practice's fringe benefits. Figure 4–3 depicts the financial aspects of the agreement.

PRACTICE INCOME		$150,000
Rent		6,345
Utilities		2,430
Salaries		29,580
Insurance		1,440
Depreciation		4,005
Professional Liability		765
Interest		1,440
Repairs		900
Legal		990
Travel		2,190
Miscellaneous		4,425
Laboratory		17,610
Drugs		480
Dental Supplies		9,000
Bad Debts		2,655
	TOTAL	84,255
	NET INCOME	$65,745

Figure 4–1 Income statement assuming $150,000 gross income (data provided by Healthco)

Gross Income		$150,000
Less Variable Expenses		
Laboratory Fees	17,610	
Drugs	480	
Dental Supplies	9,000	
Bad Debts	2,655	
TOTAL VARIABLE COST		$29,745
Less Fixed Expenses		
Rent	6,345	
Utilities	2,430	
Salaries	29,580	
Insurance	1,440	
Depreciation	4,005	
Professional Liability	765	
Interest	1,440	
Repairs	900	
Legal	990	
Travel	2,190	
Miscellaneous	4,425	
TOTAL FIXED COST		$54,510
TOTAL COSTS		$84,225
NET INCOME		$65,745

Figure 4–2 Income statement using fixed and variable cost categories

Including desired net income in the breakeven formula may seem strange to some, and while its use in the formula is not mandatory, it does give a much more complete picture of what is required to make the practice a success.

As discussed in Chapter 14, a true breakeven cannot be determined by simply adding your desired net income over and above the amount it takes to break even in the practice itself for the production of the money for the desired net income incurs additional variable costs which must be considered.

Applying the formula to the junior dentist (Figure 4–3), assume that the fixed expenses are $600 for malpractice insurance and $3,290 for social security, for a total of $3,890. The variable expense ratio will be 60 percent of the income earned, which is the percent of gross income paid to the senior dentist. Substituting the data into the breakeven formula, the junior dentist must gross $72,225 to achieve his desired net income. Assuming

$$\text{BREAKEVEN} = \frac{\text{Fixed Expense} + \text{Desired Net Income}}{(1 - \text{Variable Expense Ratio})}$$

$$= \frac{\$3{,}890 + \$25{,}000}{(1 - .60)}$$

$$= \frac{\$28{,}890}{.40}$$

$$= \$72{,}225$$

Senior Dentist Profit from Associate's Production

Senior Dentist's Share of Associate's Gross Income (.60 × $72,225)	$43,335
Less D.A. Salary	(10,000)
Less Variable Expense of Associate's Production (.20 × $72,225)	(14,445)
Senior Dentist's Profit	$18,890

Figure 4–3 Junior dentist data

that the junior dentist was successful in achieving his gross income, he would then pay the senior dentist 60 percent or $43,335.

To determine the senior dentist's profit/loss from the associateship, we subtract the additional costs he incurred as a result of the association from the $43,335. The additional costs were the $10,000 for the dental assistant plus the variable costs of the junior dentist's production, or $14,445 (.20 × $72,225). Subtracting $24,445 from the $43,335, the senior dentist's profit is $18,890.

Before leaving this subject, it is important to understand the impact of variable costs on the financial arrangements. To illustrate, let us change the terms of the agreement (Figure 4–4) to have the junior dentist pay for the dental assistant, which will increase his fixed costs from $3,890 to $13,890. Let the junior dentist also pay his own laboratory fees (which are estimated to be 12 percent of gross). The fixed expense now rises to $13,890, and the variable expense ratio changes from 60 to 72 percent (60 percent to the senior dentist plus the 12 percent laboratory fees). The junior dentist now must gross $138,893 to net his $25,000. The senior dentist now receives $83,336 from which he deducts his variable expense for the junior dentist's production (8 percent or $11,111), leaving him a net profit from the associateship of $72,225. Note that when the junior dentist paid for the dental assistant's salary, his breakeven did not increase by the $10,000 salary to $82,225, but rather it increased by $12,500 to $97,225 (as shown)

$$\text{(Breakeven} = \frac{\$13{,}890 + \$25{,}000}{(1 - .60)} = \$97{,}225)$$

because of the variable cost (40 percent) of generating the $10,000 additional ($10,000 ÷ .4 = $25,000).

Another quite common arrangement is for the junior dentist to first subtract his laboratory fees from the gross income and then pay the senior dentist a percentage of the remaining gross income. In addition, the junior is expected to pay his own laboratory fees plus the salaries and benefits of his staff. The previous breakeven formula will not work under this arrangement, but an algebraic formula can be devised as follows.

Desired net + fixed expenses = senior dentist percentage × (X − variable expense × X) − variable expense percentage × X (where X is the junior dentist's breakeven point).

To illustrate, and for comparison purposes, we will use the previous data where the junior paid for the dental assistant and a proportionate share of the laboratory fees. To this we will add paying the senior dentist a percentage of the gross equal to the senior dentist's overhead plus 10 percent (recommended by some consultants). Recall that the senior dentist's overhead was 60 percent. Substituting this data in the formula:

$$\$25{,}000 + \$13{,}890 = X - .70(X - .12X) - .12X$$
$$\$38{,}890 = X - .70X + .084X - .12X$$
$$\$38{,}890 = .264X$$
$$X = \$147{,}311$$

The junior dentist must earn $147,311 to break even. He then subtracts 12 percent ($17,677) to pay for the lab fees, leaving an adjusted gross income of $129,634. From this, 70 percent, or $90,744 is paid to the senior dentist. The senior dentist's fixed expenses by definition have not changed and the junior dentist has paid his own laboratory fees. The only expenses for which the senior dentist has not been reimbursed are the remaining variable expenses, which amount to 8 percent of the junior's gross, or $11,785. Therefore the senior realizes a net gain of $90,744 − $11,785, or $78,959 from the associateship.

While it is only good business to negotiate for a fair income, a successful associateship cannot exist if either of the two dentists is losing money. The controlling factor as to what percentage of production the jun-

$$\text{BREAKEVEN} = \frac{\text{Fixed Expense} + \text{Desired Net Income}}{(1 - \text{Variable Expense Ratio})}$$

$$= \frac{\$13{,}890 + \$25{,}000}{[1 - (.60 + .12)]}$$

$$= \frac{\$38{,}890}{.28}$$

$$= \$138{,}893$$

Senior Dentist Profit

Senior Dentist's Share of Associate's Gross Income (.60 × $138,893)..	$83,336
Less Variable Expense of Associate's Production (.08 × $138,893)	(11,111)
Senior Dentist's Profit	$72,225

Figure 4-4 Junior dentist data

ior member may receive depends on the senior dentist's variable expense ratio. A fairly reliable way to determine the *maximum* percentage that a senior dentist can afford to pay to the junior dentist is 1 − the variable expense ratio (if the senior dentist does not assume any additional fixed expenses such as dental assistant's salary). However, under this arrangement the senior dentist would normally not receive any financial benefit from the associateship.

Tax implications

It is important to determine the exact status of the associate for tax purposes. There are two possible arrangements for the associate: to work as an Independent Contractor Dentist (ICD), or as an employee. As an ICD, the associate is considered to be self-employed, which means that the associate must pay his own taxes and social security. If he is an employee, the senior dentist must withhold taxes and contribute both to social security and unemployment insurance. Regardless of what the contract says, the IRS will apply the following criteria to determine if the associate is an employee.

Does the senior dentist:

- Establish working hours, vacation time, or sick leave?
- Define the type and method of treatment?
- Restrict payment methods and specify collection policies?

44 THE ASSOCIATESHIP

- Dictate the fee schedule?
- Retain the patients if the associate leaves the practice?
- Set production goals, assign patients, select assistants, or supply laboratory materials?

If the answer to the majority of the above questions is yes, then the IRS will most likely rule that the associate is an employee.

Other considerations

- Who will pay for the professional dues and licensing?
- Will time be made available for continuing education, vacations and holidays? The minimum amount of time that both the senior dentist and the associate must devote to the practice on an annual basis should be agreed upon along with the exact date that employment begins.
- Are provisions made for buy-in to the practice and for terminating the agreement? There are at least two possible arrangements for the associateship in this respect. In one case, the senior dentist and associate are only looking for an employer/employee relationship to assist in treating the increased patient flow. Here the arrangements for the future generally specify that each will give the other a specified amount of advance notice if the contract is to be terminated.

The restrictive covenant has been mentioned in Chapter 3 and is applicable to the associateship. The restrictive covenant may also be called a "covenant not to compete." The purpose of the covenant in this case is to prevent the associate from setting up another practice close enough to affect the welfare of the senior dentist. The covenant may also contain provisions preventing the associate from working for any other dentist in the area during the period of the contract.

The legality of the covenant varies from state to state, but normally the covenant will be upheld by the court if it specifies a "reasonable distance and period of time." An excessively restrictive covenant barring the associate from practicing in the state or any contiguous state, for the lifetime of the senior dentist, probably would not be upheld by the court on the grounds that such a covenant would unduly restrict the public's access to the dental services of the associate. The ADA recommends a distance of four miles from any office of the former practice for a period of three years (see the ADA Association Agreement, Figure 4-5.)

Some consultants suggest that a portion of the associate's earnings be

EXAMPLE B: Employee Associateship Agreement

David B. Doe, D.D.S.

The following is intended to set forth our agreement with respect to your association with Dr(s). Susan L. Smith and James S. Johnson of Smith and Johnson, PA hereinafter referred to as the "Practice," with offices at 100 Main Street, Anywhere, U.S.A.

1. *Association.* You will be associated as an employee with the Practice as a general dentist on a full-time basis commencing on or about _____ _____ or at such time thereafter as you are duly licensed to practice dentistry in the State of _____. The term of your association shall be for ____ months, but either you or the Practice shall have the right to terminate your association, for any reason and without liability, upon thirty (30) days prior written notice to the other. The purpose of this association is to allow you to participate in the private practice of dentistry. The association will cease at the end of the ____ month term. If the parties wish to associate after the end of the ____ month term of this agreement, it will be necessary to execute a new written agreement.

2. *General Duties.* You will be expected to be present at the office and available for treatment of patients during general office hours. In addition, you will be expected to be available to share in the treatment of patients on weekends and in emergencies, as scheduled by the Practice.

3. *Exclusive services.* You will engage in the practice of dentistry solely as an employee of the Practice unless otherwise authorized by the Practice.

4. *Compensation.* During the ____ month period of your association, compensation will be as follows:

   The Practice will pay you for the first four months the amount of $____ ____ per month, payable ½ on the 15th of the month and ½ on the 30th of the month you commence practice.

   Beginning on the first day of the fifth month, you will be entitled to receive compensation in an amount equal to ____ percent (__%) of your gross production. Gross production for this purpose shall mean the gross fees billed for services which have been performed and completed by you, reduced by any professional or other discounts which might be granted by you or the corporation and by an amount equal to ____ percent (__%) of the laboratory charges for your production. This amount shall be computed based on your production after the last day of the fourth month through the last day covered by this agreement. Amounts due to you will be paid commencing on the fifth day of the sixth month and continuing thereafter on the fifth day of each succeeding month.

5. *Business expenses.* The Practice will pay all normal exenses including office rent, utilities and the cost of reasonable dental supplies. In addition, the Practice will furnish the following:
   1. Adequate dental equipment and instrumentation.
   2. One operatory available at all times and other operatories available by schedule.
   3. A full-time dental assistant and access to the hygiene schedule.
   4. Full support of the business office staff.

You shall obtain and pay the cost of your professional liability insurance and be responsible for ____ percent (__%) of your laboratory bill. By entering into this agreement you hereby agree to indemnify and hold Dr(s). Susan L. Smith and James S. Johnson harmless from any malpractice liability resulting from treatment provided by you.

6. *Vacations, meetings, disability pay.* You will be entitled to a total of ____ weeks per year away from the office for the purpose of vacations, professional meetings and institutes, sickness and disability. All time away from the office for all vacations and institutes shall be arranged to avoid seriously interfering with the business of the Practice and shall be taken without pay. The Practice will pay the registration fee for ____ professional meetings or continuing education seminars per year.

Figure 4–5

7. *Patient flow and management responsibilities.* The Practice will provide patients from the new patient source and from existing patients in the Practice. It is your responsibility to actively assist in securing new patients. You will attend all meetings and will be involved in all management decisions of the Practice. You will be specifically responsible for the direction of the dental assistant assigned to you.

8. *Patient records.* Your association as an employee with the Practice does not entitle you to general access to the patient records of the Practice. You shall have access only to those records of patients whom you treat.

9. *Business transactions.* You shall charge fees and collect payment in accordance with the schedule and procedures adopted by the Practice.

10. *Business records.* Your association as an employee with the Practice does not entitle you to general access to the business records of the Practice. You shall have access to the business records only to the extent necessary to verify compensation due to you from the Practice under the formula set forth in paragraph 4 of this agreement, should a dispute arise with regard thereto. Upon termination, all patient records shall remain the property of the Practice.

11. *Restrictive covenant.* In consideration of your association as an employee with the Practice, you agree that if your association is terminated for any reason by either you or the Practice, or upon lapse of time under this Agreement, you will not engage, directly or indirectly, in the practice of general dentistry whether as a proprietor, partner, employee or otherwise, within four miles of any office of the Practice in existence at the time of your termination for a period of two full years following the date of your termination. In the event that you violate the terms of this covenant not to compete, the Practice shall be entitled to obtain injunctive relief to prohibit you from such practices and obtain money damages for any injury to the Practice resulting from such competition.

12. *In case of retirement or death.* If one of the owners of the Practice should retire or die, you will be granted the first right to purchase the Practice at its fair market price to be independently determined by the average of three external appraisers to be mutually decided upon.

13. *Entire agreement amendment.* This letter of agreement includes our entire agreement with respect to your status as an employee instead of independent contractor and supersedes all oral discussions which we may have had. This agreement may be amended by you and the Practice at any time by an instrument in writing signed by both parties.

If the above properly reflects your agreement, would you please sign both copies of this letter and return one copy to the Practice.

By _____
Susan L. Smith, D.D.S., President
Smith and Johnson, Inc.

By _____
James S. Johnson, D.D.S., Vice-President
Smith and Johnson, Inc.

The above letter accurately and completely reflects our agreement with respect to my association as an employee instead of independent contractor with Susan L. Smith, D.D.S. and James S. Johnson, D.D.S. and I hereby accept this association based upon such terms and conditions.

By _____
David B. Doe, D.D.S.

Date _____

Place of Signing of Agreement _____

Attest

Building Successful Associateships, 1983, American Dental Association, Chicago.

Figure 4–5 (*Cont.*)

placed in escrow until such time as he leaves the practice and complies with the covenant. If he fails to abide by the covenant, the senior dentist receives the earnings as a form of penalty. Should the associate decide to buy into the practice, the escrow fund can then be applied toward the purchase.

The contract should specify the disposition of A/Rs produced by the associate should he leave the practice.

In the event that the senior dentist and associate are seeking a long-term relationship such as an eventual partnership, or where the senior dentist is intending to sell the practice to the associate and retire sometime in the future, the considerations become complex. The agreement should now specify how long the associate must be in the practice before he will be given an opportunity to purchase a part or all of the practice, and how the price will be determined.

Buy-sell agreement

Once the contract has been signed agreeing that the associate will one day own a part or all of the practice, the associate now has a concern about the future well-being of the practice. To prevent future problems, the contract should include provisions to protect both the associate and the senior dentist in the event that the senior dentist dies or becomes disabled.

One way of doing this is through the *buy-sell agreement,* which is a policy insuring against the death or disability of the senior dentist. The insurance policy is issued on the senior dentist with his heirs as the beneficiaries. The agreement specifies that the practice will pass to the associate upon the death or disability of the senior dentist for a stipulated price equal to that of the insurance policy. The payments for this policy are shared in a proportion to be agreed upon in the contract.

This procedure not only prevents the practice from being tied up in litigation upon the death of the senior dentist, but also specifies the value of the practice for tax purposes. Once the buy-sell agreement is backed by the insurance policy, the IRS normally will not question the price. Later, if the two dentists decide to become a partnership, a similar policy should be purchased for each dentist equal to his/her share of the practice. (See Chapter 16 for further details.)

Summary

The associateship has become an increasingly popular and viable mode of dental practice. Multiple-dentist practices can reduce fixed overhead costs and also offer the new dentist a way of starting in practice with a ready-

48 THE ASSOCIATESHIP

made patient pool and low capital investment. The associateship is not, however, without its drawbacks. Dentists seeking such an arrangement must insure that they are compatible not only from the standpoint of personality, but from philosophy of practice. The associateship agreement should be carefully negotiated in writing with the aid of an attorney. Formulas have been provided to assist in evaluating the financial implications of the agreement.

Review Questions

1. Explain how the associateship can reduce overhead as compared to a solo practice.
2. Define and discuss the use of the restrictive covenant.
3. Discuss the differences between the ICD and the employee relationship in the association.
4. Describe the tax implications and the factors that determine whether the associate is an ICD or an employee.
5. Determine the senior dentist's profit from an association based on the following data.

    The senior dentist will pay all variable expenses other than the lab fees. These expenses are estimated to be 8% of gross. The junior dentist will assume the following expenses.

    - 50% of his gross to the senior dentist
    - 12% of the gross for his lab fees
    - $12,000/year for a dental assistant
    - The junior dentist desires to gross $30,000/year

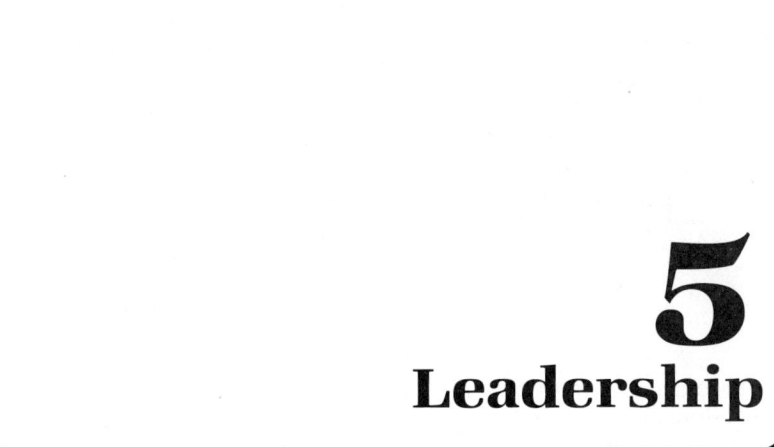

5
Leadership

Learning Objectives

Upon completion of this chapter, you should be able to:

- Discuss the difference between successful and effective leader behavior.
- Describe the levels of worker maturity and the possible leader behaviors required to increase the worker's effectiveness at each level of maturity.

Introduction

There are three skills required to be a successful manager: technical, conceptual, and human relations skills. In this chapter, we are going to discuss the human relations skills required of a successful manager, and we shall call this human relations skill *leadership*.

49

Leadership has been discussed and written about since the beginning of civilization. In earlier years, the theory was that great men possessed some unique traits which caused them to be successful in leading others. To this day writers still proclaim the "trait theory of leadership." And yet the first truly scientific research report published in 1902 described an experiment whose purpose was to determine if a leader of a group of school children would still be a leader if he were transferred to another group. The findings were that being the leader in one group did not necessarily insure that he would become a leader if transferred to another group. This indicated the possibility that leadership ability did not lie solely within the individual, but might be affected by other elements in the situation. At this writing, thousands of research reports have been written and many theories on leadership have been offered, but the truth is that very little progress has been made since that first experiment in 1902.

Leadership Research

Tracing the evolution of theory in the field of leadership will help you gain perspective regarding the problems of dealing with groups and individuals. We shall also discuss the latest theories on leadership and how they may be used to increase the effectiveness of a dental practice.

From the days of the earliest written records, writers have speculated about what caused men to become great leaders. This speculation led to many theories about the traits or attributes of leaders which caused them to become successful. Research did seem to indicate that on the whole, leaders were bigger, had more energy, and were more intelligent than the followers (but not too much more intelligent, for it led to communications problems). Nothing really concrete or applicable seemed to come from this approach, and so, in the early twentieth century, researchers began to observe the behavior of leaders in the hope that there was something unique about the way successful leaders behaved.

Several important results were reported from these studies. Ralph M. Stogdill, of Ohio State University, found that leader behavior could be divided into two independent categories: task behaviors and relations behaviors. Task behaviors are leader behaviors which concentrate on accomplishing the job, such as: encouraging the use of uniform procedures, assigning members to particular tasks, and letting members know what was expected of them. Relations behaviors are leader behaviors aimed at maintaining good relationships and morale within the group, such as: being friendly and approachable, giving the workers a say in the decisions, and doing little things to make it pleasant to be a member of the group.

When Stogdill and others at Ohio State reported these findings, many in the field of leadership assumed that leaders whose behaviors contained high amounts of both these behaviors would be the most successful leaders. Further research revealed that the "High High" leader theory was a myth, that leaders who behaved at the high end of the spectrum on both task and relations behaviors were not consistently the most successful leaders. Researchers found that in highly structured jobs where the followers had very little control over the type and pace of the work, leaders who were high in relations behaviors were the most successful. In the highly ambiguous jobs, the leader who was high in task behaviors was the most successful. Other researchers found that task-oriented leaders had more productive groups in the short run but higher grievance rates and more turnover in the long run. It has also been reported that there is an area of indifference among followers relating to the extremes of behavior in both task and relations orientation. In other words, for each group there is an optimum level of task and relations behavior.

As this line of research progressed, it became apparent that the success of the leader depended not only upon his own behavior, but also upon the fit between the demands of the job setting and the leader's behavior. As the leadership research became more sophisticated, it was reported that not only was there an interaction between the job setting and the leader's behavior as it affected group satisfaction, productivity and turnover, but also that the personality and past experience of the worker must be entered into the equation. For example, workers who had authoritarian personalities responded better to task behaviors than they did to relations behaviors.

It has also been reported that various personality traits affect not only the leader behaviors that the followers want, but also affect the followers' perceptions of the leader's behavior. Still later, researchers have found that the leader's predisposition to these leader behaviors (leadership style) is affected in turn by the leader's personality and past experiences.

These findings have culminated in what is now termed the *contingency theory* of leadership. In its simplest form this theory states that the effectiveness of a leader's behavior will depend upon the situation.

Figure 5-1 illustrates the contingency theory as follows. The interaction between the leader and the follower(s) is circular. The leader emits a leadership behavior that is based upon his past experience in reaction to his perception of the situation, which is in turn distorted to an extent by his personality. The leader's reaction is also affected by organizational con-

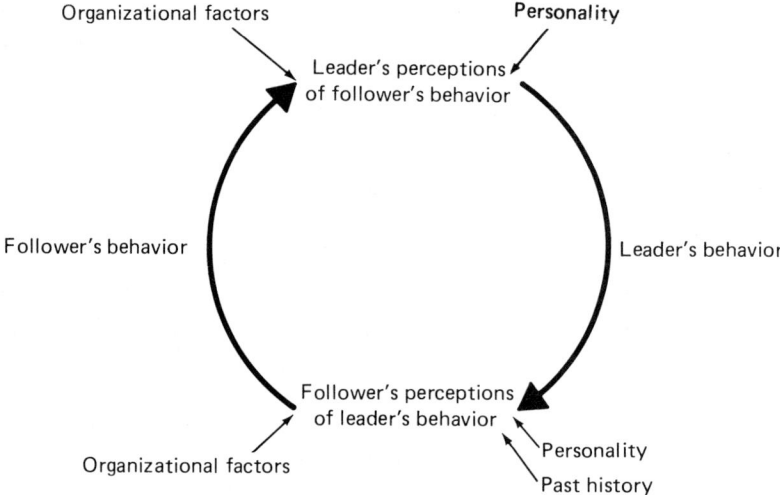

Figure 5-1 Leader and follower perceptions of each others' behavior.

straints. For example, few organizations would permit the leader to resort to physical violence to carry out his job. There are also likely to be operating procedures and legislation that restrict the amount of authority the leader may delegate to his subordinates.

Considering these restraints and his perception of the situation, the leader emits a behavior which is observed and interpreted by the follower(s) depending upon their past experience and personality traits. As in the case of the leader, the response behavior by the follower(s) is affected by the organizational constraints in existence. The leader observes and interprets the behavior of the follower(s), and the cycle is repeated.

The Hersey/Blanchard Theory of Leadership

The theory which we are going to describe is taken from the book *Management of Organizational Resources*, by Paul Hersey and Ken Blanchard, which bases its leadership approach largely on the research we have just discussed.

Definitions

First, we must clarify the definition of leadership. Leadership is simply trying to influence others to do what you want them to do and is not confined to the workplace, but comes into play in your dealings with friends, children, and spouses. It exists any time you attempt to influence others to engage in some behavior designed to achieve your goal(s).

There is, however, an important distinction to be made between *successful* and *effective* leadership as illustrated in Figure 5–2. When person A attempts to influence person B to act, the degree of successful leadership is measured by the degree to which B complies with the request. While compliance is a necessary precondition for effective leadership, a leader can be successful and yet not be effective. The effectiveness of the leader is determined by the degree to which the leader's directions to B helped to attain the leader's goal. For example, under these definitions, we must say that Hitler was a successful leader in that he was able to influence the majority of the German people to do what he wished, but he was not an effective leader in that he failed to achieve his goal of world domination.

Hersey and Blanchard maintain that effective leadership is attained when you, as the leader, are able to vary the blend of relations and task behaviors to meet the maturity of your subordinate(s) so that they are motivated to work to achieve your goals. We have already defined relations and task behaviors and also talked about situations in which these behaviors were effective or ineffective. There are two dimensions to an individual's maturity: psychological maturity, which affects the willingness to do a job, and task maturity, which is the ability to accomplish a task. There are four possible combinations of these two maturity dimensions.

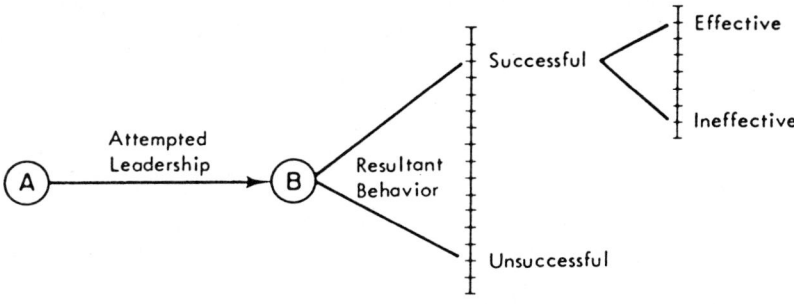

Paul Hersey/Kenneth H. Blanchard, *Management of Organization Behavior: Utilizing Human Resources*, 4th ed., © 1982, pp. 110, 262. Reprinted by permission of Prentice-Hall, Inc., Englewood Cliffs, N. J.

Figure 5–2 Successful and effective leadership continuums

1. Unwilling and unable
2. Unable and willing
3. Able but unwilling
4. Willing and able

The lowest maturity level is the worker who is both unable and unwilling to do a job. The next level of maturity is the worker who is unable but willing. Still more mature is the individual who is able but unwilling, and finally, the highest level of maturity exists in the person who is both willing and able.

The Theory

It is also important to recognize that these maturity combinations may vary within the individual depending upon the task. It is not unusual to find a dental assistant who is very mature when she is chairside assisting, but who is very immature when it comes to handling the supply inventory. It is important to assess an individual's maturity level on individual tasks, and not to assign and respond to an overall maturity level.

In Figure 5-3, Hersey and Blanchard have combined individual maturity levels with the recommended leader behavior as indicated by the bell-shaped curve drawn across the four quadrants. From this illustration, you can see that the behavior with the highest probability of being effective for the lowest maturity level (quadrant 1), unwilling and unable, is a combination of high task and low relationship. In this case, you are engaging in a predominantly one-way communication with the staff member, telling her exactly what to do and how to do it and then supervising closely to see that she complies.

If you are successful in increasing the maturity level of your staff member to the point where she is now willing but not yet able to perform an assigned task, she has now moved to quadrant 2 where high task and high relations behaviors on your part are likely to be the most effective. As the maturity of the individual increases still further, your blend of task and relations behaviors will change to high relations and low task (quadrant 3), and then to both low relations and low task as the worker reaches the highest level of maturity (quadrant 4). It is your responsibility as the leader to develop your staff so that they can reach the highest level of maturity possible consistent with your skill as a leader and their particular combination of personality and skills.

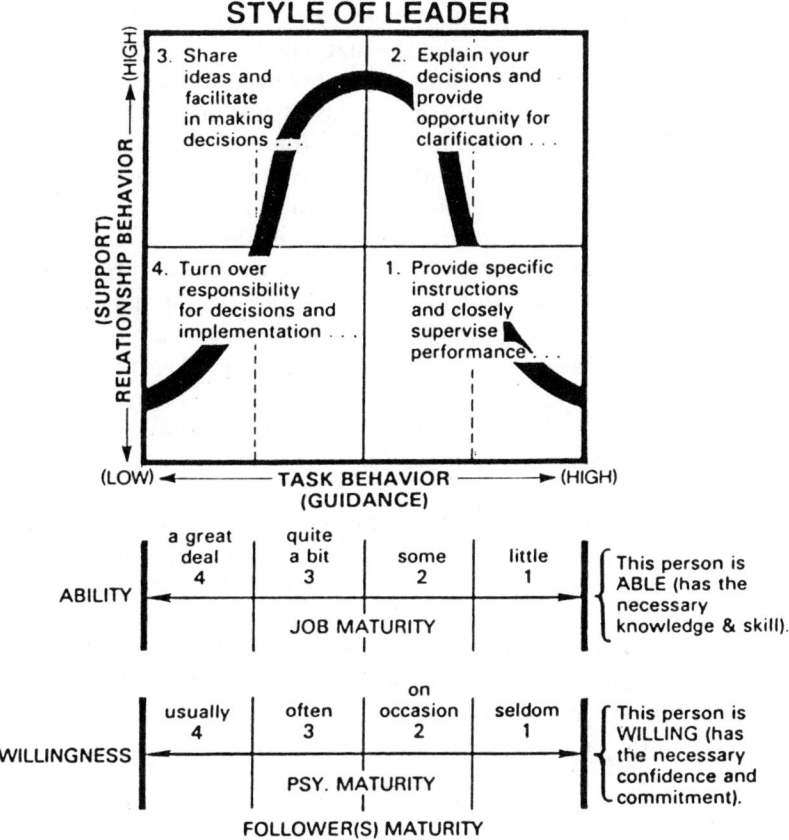

Paul Hersey/Kenneth H. Blanchard, *Management of Organizational Behavior: Utilizing Human Resources*, 4th ed., © 1982, pp. 110, 262. Reprinted by permission of Prentice-Hall, Inc., Englewood Cliffs, N.J.

Figure 5-3

Your ability to be an effective leader and to increase the maturity of your staff members depends upon your ability to correctly assess the maturity level of your worker, or the work group, and your ability to behave in the manner required. Earlier in this chapter, we discussed how personality can distort your perceptions of the behavior of others. If you have an authoritarian personality, you will most frequently assess your followers as immature and thus justify the authoritarian behaviors characterized by the high task, low relations behaviors in quadrant 1.

Because of our culture and a natural desire to be liked, the majority of Americans tend to be limited in their ability to operate in quadrant 1.

They have a tendency to be either high relations and high task, or high relations and low task. Fortunately, the maturity level of the average American worker results in the optimum leader behaviors being in either quadrant 2 or 3. When consultants tried to instill the high relations style of management into a pajama factory in India, the managers became ineffective, because the maturity level and the culture of the Indian people called for authoritarian (quadrant 1) leader behavior.

Most leaders also seem to resist the low relations, low task behaviors of quadrant 4, apparently feeling that the best leaders are those who interact the most with their followers. They operate well in quadrant 3 with its high relations, low task requirements, but they can't let go of the idea that their people must depend upon them for psychological support. Actually, the mature worker typical of quadrant 4 derives her rewards from the nature of the work itself and has the confidence and ability to know when she is performing well and so does not need the support of her supervisor.

The key to effective leader behavior, then, is the ability to correctly assess the maturity level of your staff. This requires control of the biases which distort perception, and also an awareness of the cues which can tell you when the follower's maturity changes. In addition, you must have the will and self-discipline to be able to vary your behavior across the four quadrants as required. The only other alternative is to increase your skills to the point where you can successfully identify and hire staff members who require your particular mode of leader behavior.

Theory Application

To illustrate the application of this theory, assume you have just hired a new dental assistant. On the first day, you schedule her to polish amalgams on a patient. You notice that she is very reluctant to accept the task, taking an unusually long time to get set up, and when you examine the finished amalgams, you find that the polishes have been done very poorly.

In analyzing the situation using our theory, you would probably determine from observation that she was not willing to do the polishes and you could assume from the unsatisfactory polishes that she also lacked the skill to do the job properly. If her failure to accomplish the job was due to her lack of motivation, the reason for this lack of motivation should be determined. There are two possible reasons for her lack of motivation: (1) she doesn't like to do polishes and finds the task unrewarding, or (2) she lacks the skill to do the polishes properly and thus feels insecure for she knows that you will be displeased with the end results of her efforts.

In the case of her disliking the task, you must decide if it is important that she do polishes as part of her duties. If it is important, you must then insist that she do polishes when requested or be terminated. (It is very important that you fully outline the duties of the job during the hiring interview so that the request that an assistant do polishes when scheduled should be no surprise.) If she cannot be motivated to do polishes and do them well, she should be terminated without delay.

If you find that the lack of motivation is caused by a lack of skill, you will need to conduct a training program to impart those skills to your dental assistant. The leader behaviors required during the initial phase of the training should be the low relations, high task behaviors of quadrant 1. In the beginning, the conversation will be mostly one-way, from you to the assistant, as you explain and demonstrate the procedures required to polish an amalgam. As the training proceeds, the conversation will become more of a two-way conversation as the assistant begins to ask and answer questions. As she progresses, you will start increasing the amount of relations behaviors by complimenting her on her progress and rewarding her by permitting her to accomplish more and more of the procedure on her own.

You will eventually move into quadrant 2 with the high relations, high task behaviors as she becomes more and more competent at this particular task. You will slowly reduce the amount of your task behaviors as she becomes proficient and ceases to require the close supervision and instruction.

As your assistant grows more competent, you will move to quadrant 3, with high relations and low task behaviors. Continued instruction in polishing will now be demotivating, since she will think you are talking down to her. Her motivation is kept high by positive feedback, compliments, smiles, or bonuses as her performance continues to improve. Finally, you will slowly decrease your positive feedback until your behaviors become the low task, low relations behaviors of quadrant 4. The assistant now knows her job and receives her rewards from knowing when she has done a good job.

I think a word of caution is required here. I personally have found that very few people ever reach the quadrant 4 level of maturity to the degree that positive feedback is not required to keep them motivated.

There is no known way to accurately determine the maturity level of a subordinate. The only practical way of finding the optimum blend of behaviors is through trial and error and close observation. Keeping in mind the practical and ethical requirement to keep developing the maturity of your staff, you must try moving them along the bell curve of Figure 5-3 from quadrant 1 toward quadrant 4 in a series of small steps.

For example, as you move an auxiliary through quadrant 1 to quadrant 2, you should increase positive feedback and grant more autonomy in small increments. If performance improves, repeat the process. If performance does not improve, it is an indication that you have overestimated her maturity and must move back along the curve by slightly increasing task behavior and slightly decreasing relations behavior.

There will be occasions when your auxiliary's performance will decrease, requiring you to move in the direction of quadrant 1. For example, a dental assistant whose performance is typical of the quadrant 3 maturity level may become forgetful and distracted in the performance of her duties, perhaps because of problems outside the office. In this case, you would move toward quadrant 2 in a series of small steps, increasing your task behaviors and decreasing your relations behaviors until the performance degradation ceases, and then start over again from that position to work your assistant back toward quadrant 4 in a series of small steps.

It will help if you describe the theory to your staff and explain how their behavior, or maturity level, determines your behavior. Those who wish to be treated in a manner characterized by quadrant 3 and not be treated in a manner characterized by quadrant 1, for example, must develop the skills and willingness characteristic of the quadrant 3 maturity level.

Summary

This has been a brief discussion of the leadership theories and a demonstration of the theory that I feel has the most practical application. While the theory may be far from perfect, it does present a framework from which to develop your leadership ability. However, no theory will work unless you develop self-control, a sense of responsibility for the development of those who work with you, and a sense of awareness of their feelings and needs.

Nothing I have said here is intended to suggest that your responsibility for your patients is to be subordinated to the needs of your staff. Your first responsibility is to your patients. After that, your next responsibility is toward those who work with you. Any staff member who detracts from your primary responsibility and will not progress to a level of competency, despite coaching and feedback using the methods we have discussed, must be terminated.

Review Questions

1. Explain the difference between successful and effective leader behaviors.
2. Define the two major leader behaviors.
3. Describe the maturity level applicable to Hersey/Blanchard's four quadrants in terms of ability and motivation. Then describe the leader behavior combination that would have the highest probability of success for each of the maturity levels.

6
Communication in a Dental Practice

Learning Objectives

Upon completion of this chapter, you should be able to:

- Conduct effective staff meetings.
- Discuss the uses of the various communication methods available in a dental practice.
- Discuss the importance of non-evaluative feedback.

Introduction

Once you have located your practice and recruited the members of your dental staff, you are ready to start treating patients. However, at this point all your objectives, policies, and procedures are known only to you. Now you are faced with the question, "How am I to inform my staff of my objectives, policies, plans and procedures?" Not only must you insure that your subordinates know your desires in this respect, you also must motivate them to actively accept and effectively work for the attainment of these objectives.

It is also reasonable to assume that your policies, procedures and objectives will require modification from time to time to cope with problems that arise. To operate an effective dental practice you must become aware of the problems early, before they can seriously affect your practice.

To insure that your objectives, policies, and procedures become a reality, you must:

- Select a method to communicate your objectives, policies, and procedures to your staff.
- Recognize problems early and take necessary corrective action before the problems have a chance to affect your practice.
- Decide when and what problems should be discussed with your staff to reach quality decisions and to motivate the staff to accept those decisions.

Ways of Communicating

What are some of the ways you can communicate with your staff? Probably the first thought that comes to your mind is, "I don't see any problem. I have such a small staff that I can easily just tell them what I want as we work." There are a few problems with this seemingly simple approach. First, there are few people who can do two things at once. If you try to pass on your objectives, policies, and procedures while attending to the day-to-day duties, probably much of what you tell your subordinates will be lost through their inattention. Second, you will soon find that you forget to tell all of your staff about some important policy or decision. It is very easy to lose track of whom you have talked to while trying to treat patients. Third, you will find that your subordinates will not always understand a statement which to you is perfectly clear.

Despite the serious drawbacks of this means of communication, there are certain advantages. Particularly in a small dental practice, oral communications have the advantages of being fast, requiring minimum effort, and providing for the all-important feedback required for ensuring understanding and motivation.

After you have realized that this means of communicating with your staff leaves much to be desired, you might decide to simply choose one of your staff members and give her the responsibility of passing the word to the others. This method has two major drawbacks. First, you must be very certain that the individual you choose fully understands your message and can pass it on without distortion — a very unlikely possibility. You will find that each individual has built-in filters which cause them to interpret messages based upon their past experience and personality. In most cases the reinterpretation loses much of the original message.

Second, you must be aware of the group dynamics impact of selecting another individual as your spokesman. That person may well gain an unintended increase in status because the other staff members are likely to perceive that you have given that person a leadership position in your practice. Such an inadvertent action may lead the other members of the staff to resent this new leader and thus seriously impair the effectiveness of your team.

If you decide to use one of your staff as a supervisor in this sense, be sure that you make an announcement of the fact to the rest of the staff along with a clear delineation of her responsibilities and authority. If you disregard this advice because of your confidence in the person you chose for this responsibility, remember that it will be difficult for her to overcome staff resentment and establish her authority without this announcement. This method of communication shares some of the advantages of the previous communications method in that it is fast and requires a minimum amount of effort. However, unlike the previous method, it does not provide for the all-important feedback and is subject to distortion.

Still another approach to the communications problem is to use written memos and the office manual to disseminate your objectives, policies, and procedures. These two means of communication are absolutely essential and will certainly improve the dissemination of information to your staff. Using memos insures that everyone receives exactly the same information, and using the office manual provides a permanent source of guidance to your staff as to your objectives, policies, and procedures.

However, when used alone, these methods have deficiencies. First, it is an unusual individual who can consistently express his thoughts clearly and concisely in writing. Second, and related, is the lack of a means of feedback from your staff to ensure that they are correctly interpreting and completely understand your message. Third, this method is time consuming for you, the writer.

All the previous means of communications leave something to be desired in insuring that the message is received and understood. More seriously, used by themselves, these methods either fail to transmit an accurate message or fail to provide a means of feedback to ensure that the message is understood. Equally, if not more, important is the fact that these methods do not assist you in motivating your staff to accept and actively support your objectives.

What has been missing from these previous methods is the opportunity for direct face-to-face exchange of ideas with your people without the distractions of the day-to-day operations.

Staff Meetings

Staff meetings can be one of the most effective means of coordinating, directing, and motivating your staff. The staff meeting provides you with an uninterrupted, organized means of interacting with your staff for the sole purpose of determining the best means of improving the effectiveness of the practice. By uninterrupted, I mean that a specific time and place should be set aside for this purpose and that all other operations be suspended so that you and your staff can concentrate on the meeting without interruption by telephone calls or any other business. It is a time for you and your staff to gain perspective and greater insight into the practice.

In the staff meeting you may communicate your objectives, policies, and procedures, and through frank and open discussion, you have the opportunity to gain the feedback necessary to insure that your staff understands what you expect from them. This meets the first problem of effectively disseminating objectives, policies, and procedures.

The staff meeting provides the time for you and your people to review your operation and discover potential problem areas. In the meeting you should review the progress toward the objectives you have set through management by objectives. By setting specific, measurable, time-oriented objectives, you have a means of determining progress toward those objectives and early identification of problems which may hinder their attainment.

Remember the considerations of quality, acceptance, and time in deciding what problems to bring to your staff. (See Chapter 9.) Nothing can be more demotivating to your staff than to ask them to participate in the decision-making when you already have your own solution to the problem and will not be willing to accept their recommendations.

Equally important if you really want their unbiased solutions to a problem is the manner in which you conduct the meeting. You must avoid leading the staff to your solution. This means that your role during the problem solving must be that of a facilitator whose task is to keep the discussion moving by asking for clarification and insuring that each member has an opportunity to contribute to the process.

Team building

You and your assistants operate in a unique environment characterized by close physical proximity for sustained periods of time. This environment places unusual demands on the dental team. In most other professions, if the leader is having an "off day" when he just does not feel up to interacting with subordinates, he can normally resort to other activities such as planning or routine paperwork which do not require close association with others. With you and your assistants, even if one of you is experiencing an "off day," you must still associate with each other in a very confined space.

This unusual situation necessitates that you and your assistants develop close, supporting relationships characterized by a frank and open exchange of job-relevant feelings. Such relationships can be developed through effective staff meetings.

Each staff meeting should devote time to developing a rapport among the members of the dental team. This does not mean that staff meetings are to be turned into sensitivity training sessions. The privacy of the individual must be respected. A sensitive dentist must be aware of the personal problems of his individual staff members — but he should not attempt to probe into their personal lives except as a last resort, and then not in a staff meeting but in private, and then only when the personal problems of the member are interfering with the effectiveness of the practice.

Team building is an important element of any small group; thus, it is applicable to the usual dental practice. *Team building* means developing an ability within the group to exchange frank, open, non-evaluative feedback on task-relevant matters. *Non-evaluative feedback* is feedback which describes the behavior of another and how that behavior makes you feel. Non-evaluative feedback does not attempt to attribute reasons for the individual's behavior, or attempt to evaluate the person based upon their behavior. *Task-relevant behaviors* are those behaviors that have an effect on job performance. Never criticize or offer evaluative feedback to a team member at the staff meeting or in the presence of others. Such public criticism threatens the individual's self-image and will almost always create deep and long-lasting resentment.

For example, it would be appropriate for an assistant to offer the comment that you appear to be so engrossed in the treatment that you fail to establish rapport with the patients (non-evaluative feedback). It would not be appropriate to comment that you do not establish rapport with the patients because you do not care about their well-being. This second comment is evaluative feedback which attacks your self-image.

Similarly, it might be appropriate for you to comment that your staff is not operating effectively in getting the first patient seated in the morning.

It would not be appropriate for you to say that the reason for the problem is that one of your assistants is dating too much and therefore is both late getting to the office in the morning and too tired to work effectively once she gets there. This might be a subject for private discussion with the assistant, but even then it would be best to limit the conversation to the fact that she has developed a habit of being late and does not perform effectively. The reason for the problem is for her to determine and correct. If she is unable to correct the deficiency after sufficient counseling, she may then be asked to leave the practice.

Implementing the staff meeting program

Now that we have looked at what the staff meeting is supposed to accomplish, what is the best way to implement an effective staff meeting program? I have already discussed the importance of setting aside an uninterrupted period of time for the staff meeting.

Equally important is the timing of the staff meeting. You should set a consistent schedule, such as every Thursday at 1:00 PM, and stick to this schedule even if you have nothing of major importance to discuss. Unless you and your staff develop a habit of preparing for and attending the staff meetings at a set time, your staff will most likely forget and you will lose time trying to get them together. It is also very frustrating for your staff to have to keep asking each other if there will be a staff meeting today. Even if you have nothing to say, get your staff together at the specified time, ask for any last-minute problems, and dismiss them. In the long run you will save time by being consistent with your schedule.

When you first start your practice, or when you have had a large change in your staff, you will probably need to have a weekly staff meeting to disseminate your objectives, policies and procedures and to amend them as you gain experience. As the staff becomes more coordinated, you may wish to schedule staff meetings less frequently, however, with a large staff, I strongly recommend having a meeting at least twice a month to insure that you are continuing in your motivation and team building efforts.

With a new staff, the staff meeting will serve as a means of getting your staff acquainted with one another. A word of advice here: Don't be surprised if the first several meetings appear to be ineffective. During these first few meetings your staff will not be paying much attention to the practical aspects of the practice.

Typically, all groups go through several phases in their development. In the first phase the individual members are more concerned about finding their place in the group. Much of the informal discussion will focus on establishing commonalities and differences. Each will be seeking for things they have in common with the others, such as where they went to school, mutual acquaintances, and the possible similarities in values. Each will be determining how much of herself it is safe to reveal and how much status and power she will have in the group. Only after the individual members have found a comfortable relationship in the group will they be ready to consider other factors such as how to go about getting the job done. Remember to allow time for the group to form before trying to get down to business.

Time is money, and an ineffective staff meeting is a prime waster of time. The effectiveness of your staff meeting depends in large part upon the use of an agenda. Over time, you will find that the agenda becomes fairly well fixed and changes very little. A typical example of an agenda follows.

1. Dissemination of new objectives, procedures, and information
2. Discussion of possible problem areas
    a. patient management
    b. financial
    c. supply
    d. general administration
    e. interpersonal problems
3. Individual progress reports on assigned projects
4. Consideration of new projects
5. Evaluation of staff meeting
6. Summary of staff meeting

The use of an agenda provides a means of progressing through the staff meeting in an orderly, organized manner. There will probably be times when you must diplomatically steer the discussion back to the agenda since your staff will tend to wander in their discussions, but in time they will learn to appreciate this organized approach. It will also speed up the staff meeting process if you distribute a copy of the agenda to each member a few days before the meeting. This allows them time to think about the problems proposed in the agenda and any other contributions they may want to make. By jotting notes on the agenda, they will be better prepared to make a meaningful contribution. You may also wish to set up a procedure so that your staff can make suggestions for items to be included in the agenda.

While proper use of the agenda permits effective use of the meeting time, you must avoid dominating the meeting so that the staff will feel free to indulge in frank discussions of task-relevant problems. The dentist who takes the role of the teacher or autocrat and simply disseminates his policies in a running stream of conversation, ending with "any comments" and then closes the meeting is denying himself the benefits of the staff's knowledge.

Many dentists try to be overly efficient. They arrive and start the meeting promptly by reading from prepared notes. I have observed dentists who were so absorbed in reading their notes that they failed to observe their staff's reactions. For example, they announced a new policy by reading directly from their notes, only to miss the raised eyebrows and facial expressions of dismay that passed between the staff members. When they did glance up from their notes, the staff members had regained their composure and the dentist had no inkling of their feelings about the new policy. He later wondered why the new policy was ineffective. A skilled leader would have kept his eyes on the staff members and, catching their expressions, would have invited comments which may have led to a modification or even a changed policy which would have succeeded because it was accepted by the staff.

Many times a dentist really tries to enlist the comments of his staff but only listens superficially. For example, during a recent staff meeting an auxiliary, smiling slightly, commented that she didn't feel that the dentist was equitably delegating the more challenging dental procedures because she had been assigned to polishing amalgams most of the previous week. Misled by her smiling, soft-spoken comment, the dentist merely smiled back and turned to discuss the next item on the agenda. At the end of the meeting, I asked him if he had heard the auxiliary's comments. His reply indicated that he had, but hadn't thought it particularly important. A little more probing of the auxiliary revealed that she was really unhappy about what she considered a lack of confidence in her ability. She further admitted that if such a condition continued, she would probably look for another job.

If you have a staff that is truly dedicated to attaining the goals of your practice, there will be times when differences of opinion will arise during the decision-making process. While your staff may agree on the goal to be attained, there may be serious disagreements as to the best means of attaining the goal. These disagreements will place you, as the leader, in the difficult position of attempting to resolve the conflict without demotivating some of your staff.

Some will try to take the easy way out by putting the decision to a vote without taking the time to ensure that each of the staff has an opportunity to be heard. When you submit the decision to a vote prematurely, you may be setting up a *win-lose situation,* meaning that the majority in the vote are the winners and the minority are the losers. Researchers have found that such situations tend to cause long-lasting resentment on the part of the losers and a need to maintain the top hand on the part of the winners. While neither the winners nor the losers may be aware of their feelings, this split over issues may well carry over for years so that the staff will unconsciously polarize into the same two competing groups every time a decision is required. While a vote may at times be unavoidable, it may be possible to avoid this polarization by insuring that each member feels that he has a chance to make his position clear and that that position was respected even if the others could not accept it.

A word of caution is appropriate here. If you pride yourself on the lack of conflict in your staff meetings, consider two unpleasant possibilities. First, if may be that your staff is just not motivated and doesn't care about the objectives of the practice. In this case, they have nothing at stake and probably feel that contributing to the discussion is just too much effort — better to just relax and let the boss worry about the problems. Or, second, they may be afraid of you. After all, you control their means of livelihood. If they feel that you will retaliate against any disagreement, they are unlikely to risk disagreeing with you. Fear and lack of motivation are the two most serious detractors from effective communications in a work setting.

Telling your staff members that you want to know about their feelings on task-relevant matters is usually not enough, since there will be a certain amount of reticence among them. Developing an atmosphere of mutual trust within your staff may take years of patient encouragement and self-control on your part. When you have reason to believe that the staff is not being open with you, you must probe gently and diplomatically until you are reasonably sure that you have correctly understood their feelings. If you become impatient or lose your temper, you can lose their confidence and have to start from zero once again to regain their trust.

Item five (evaluation of the staff meeting) on the staff meeting agenda mentioned previously is particularly important to the team building process. In evaluating the staff meeting, you should examine whether or not the staff felt that the meeting gave them ample opportunity to participate, if the climate of the meeting contributed to frank and open discussion, if the agenda was adequate, and how efficiently the meeting was conducted.

The use of the summary at the end of the meeting is also essential to insure that the staff leave the meeting with the key points of the discussion firmly in their minds and that all are clear on exactly what decisions were made. I recommend that you jot down short notes to remind yourself of the key decisions made as the meeting progresses and at the end of the meeting quickly review the major points to insure understanding by both you and your staff.

As you go over your summary, you will be surprised at how often your staff misinterpret your decisions. Equally important is the necessity of assigning one of the staff the responsibility for incorporating the new policies into the office manual. If this is not done, the same decisions will have to be made over again in a few months when you and your staff forget the decisions that have been made.

One last recommendation is that you hold a *stand-up meeting* every morning. I call this a stand-up meeting because no one sits down. It is amazing how short a meeting can become when people have to remain standing. In this meeting, you and your staff should review the plans for the day's operation including a thorough review of the patients' health records and the specific treatments to be rendered for each patient on the schedule. This will protect the patient who requires premedication or who has contraindications in the health record. It will also help you avoid embarrassing situations such as seating the patient and then realizing you have misplaced the treatment plan, or finding that the patient's partial has not been delivered from the laboratory.

Summary

Communications can be a serious problem even in a small-group operation like the dental office. The staff meeting is an excellent management tool if used properly, since it will help you to communicate with the staff and thus coordinate the team's efforts, provide feedback on performance, and help you to utilize the talents of your staff to improve the effectiveness of your practice. As leaders, dentists must be aware of the implications of evaluative feedback and the importance of developing mutual trust through team building.

Review Questions

1. What type of communications provides the best feedback?
2. Describe the use of the agenda in the staff meeting.
3. Should you encourage dissent in your staff meetings, and if so, why?

7
Small Group Dynamics

Learning Objectives

Upon completion of this chapter, you should be able to:

- Discuss how individuals differ in their needs and how the group and your behavior can help to meet these needs.
- Discuss how group norms and cohesiveness can interact to affect group productivity.
- Discuss how to identify and cope with interpersonal conflict.

Introduction

As a dentist you will find that an understanding of small group dynamics will make it possible for you to increase the effectiveness of your dental team. By applying the theories of group dynamics, you can obtain desirable behavior from your team members.

A dental team has certain unique characteristics. It is a group whose members work in close physical proximity, have very similar training, and in which successful performance of the team requires a high degree of cooperation since each member is dependent upon the others for successful completion of their tasks.

The nature of this group provides both advantages and disadvantages as it applies to stress and group effectiveness. The group's small size increases the individual's feelings of belonging and importance because group interaction and communications are both encouraged and facilitated. The disadvantage is that the team members must work in close proximity and are very interdependent, so that the actions of one member have an impact on the success and satisfaction of the others. The potential for interpersonal conflict in such a close working relationship is very high.

Group Characteristics

To better understand the group dynamics, let us look at some of the characteristics of the group. First, why do people join groups? Research indicates that people join groups for a variety of reasons, all of which serve to fulfill some individual need. Some of the reasons people join groups are:

- They are attracted to the goals of the group.
- They like the activities that take place in the group.
- They have a need to affiliate with others.
- They believe that joining the group will increase their status.
- They value the achievement and challenge provided by the group.
- They join work groups to earn money with which they can fulfill still other needs.

It is quite probable that each individual is fulfilling some of the needs to some degree. But for every individual, the strength of these needs varies and forms a unique combination characterizing the individual. Therefore, you must treat each individual differently in recognition of these various needs. For example, the auxiliary who joins your team to fulfill a need for affiliation will probably respond more readily to opportunities to interact with you and the other auxiliaries than she will to such things as an increase in pay. An auxiliary who joins the group because of a high need for achievement is not as interested in the interpersonal interactions as she is in the challenge of high performance standards.

Group cohesiveness

One of the major dimensions in group dynamics is group cohesiveness. Group cohesiveness is defined as the sum of all forces acting on a group member to remain in the group and the degree to which the reasons for joining the group are met. In other words, group cohesiveness is the strength of the attractiveness of such things as group goals, group activities, the need for affiliation, status, and achievement.

Just what does group cohesiveness do in the group? Highly cohesive groups are characterized by a higher level of personal interaction and communications between their members. The members also have a higher opinion of themselves and of the group. Group cohesiveness reduces the workers' anxiety and increases job satisfaction. This in turn lowers absenteeism and turnover, all other things being equal. While it is true that absenteeism and turnover are very serious considerations in the effective operation of your practice, high group cohesiveness does not necessarily increase the group's effectiveness in obtaining your practice goals. We shall see why shortly.

You must also remember that the auxiliary is constantly comparing the cost of belonging to the group with other alternatives. When an auxiliary joins your group, she is choosing to work for you in preference to other activities such as being a mother, being with friends, playing bridge, or working for someone else. She is also comparing the amount of effort that she is putting into her job with the rewards she receives such as her pay, recognition, and the attractiveness of her co-workers. Having considered these, she looks at the other alternatives available, and if these alternatives are more attractive, she will leave your group for the alternatives.

The important point is that because an auxiliary stays with your team does not mean that she is particularly satisfied. It merely means that she does not perceive any alternative which is more attractive. For example, a recent research project found that the workers on the job were very dissatisfied with their pay, yet they did not leave the organization because in a period of business recession, they did not perceive any alternative that would be more attractive.

Group norms

The next important dimension to consider is group norms, which are the generally agreed-upon standards of behavior for the group members that have emerged as a consequence of member interaction over time. These standards are normally unwritten, and in fact, the members may not be conscious that such standards exist. However, be assured that these norms do have a major effect on the behavior of the individual group members in your dental practice.

These norms vary widely among groups. They may cover such areas as dress, behavior, productivity, and cooperativeness. Norms may be considered either pivotal or peripheral. A pivotal norm is one that the group considers to be absolutely essential and with which its members must comply. Failure of a group member to comply with a pivotal norm may result in her ejection or isolation from the group. One of the pivotal norms might be that when one of the auxiliaries in the group isn't busy she assist the other auxiliaries who are working. Should one of the auxiliaries fail to meet this standard, she will come under the group sanctions which we shall discuss in a moment.

A peripheral norm is behavior which the group considers to be beneficial but not absolutely necessary. A common example might be that the practice members prefer to wear slacks, but would not be upset if one of the members wore a skirt (assuming the member is female, of course). "Good" group members (in the eyes of the group) are expected to adopt these norms as their personal values.

Table 7-1 indicates some of the possible norms that could be held by your staff. Note that there are positive and negative norms. Those that are congruent with your practice goals are naturally the ones you will consider the positive norms. Those that are detrimental to the achievement of your goals will be considered negative norms. It should be obvious from the examination of this chart that norms are critical to effective operation of your team practice. This leads to the question of how and why groups develop negative norms and what you as a dentist can do about it.

Research indicates that negative group norms develop when the group members feel that they are being treated unfairly (that is, if they feel underpaid and overworked, if they don't foresee that they are receiving status that they feel entitled to, if they fail to receive adequate recognition, and/or if they feel that they are not being treated as individuals of worth). You as a manager must be aware of these causes and strive to reduce the possibility of negative norm development.

Now that we understand a little about the nature of the two major dimensions, group cohesiveness and group norms, let us see how they interact to affect group effectiveness. Research indicates that highly cohesive groups are far more likely to enforce the norms than groups low in cohesiveness. They enforce these norms through communications, threats, withholding of recognition, withholding of affiliation, and in extreme cases, ejection of the member from the group.

When your staff perceives that one of your auxiliaries is deviating from

Table 7-1 Categories of organizational norms with possible positive and negative examples

Categories	Examples of positive norms	Examples of negative norms
Organizational and personal pride	Auxiliaries speak for the practice when it is criticized unfairly	Auxiliaries don't care about practice problems
Performance/excellence	Auxiliaries try to improve, even if they are doing well	Auxiliaries are satisfied with the minimum level of performance necessary
Teamwork/communication	Auxiliaries listen and are receptive to the ideas and opinions of others	Auxiliaries gossip behind the backs of others rather than deal with issues openly and constructively
Leadership/supervision	Auxiliaries ask for help when they need it	Auxiliaries hide their problems and avoid the dentist
Colleague/associate relations	Auxiliaries refuse to take advantage of fellow auxiliaries	Auxiliaries don't care about the well-being of others on the team
Customer/consumer relations	Auxiliaries show concern about serving the patients	Auxiliaries are indifferent and, when possible, hostile to patients
Honesty and security	Auxiliaries are concerned about dishonesty and pilferage	Auxiliaries are expected to steal a little and be honest only when necessary
Training and development	Auxiliaries really show they care about training and development	There is much talk about training and development but no one takes it seriously
Innovation and change	Auxiliaries are usually looking for better ways of doing their jobs	Auxiliaries stick to the old ways of doing their jobs

the norms, the first overt symptom is usually increased communications between the other members of the team and the deviant auxiliary. The group will seek to convince her of the rightness of the group norm. If this persuasion is not successful, you will then note that during the coffee break the deviant is no longer included in the group, nor is she apt to be invited to lunch with the other women. Having failed to persuade this auxiliary to accept the norms, the team will now see her as a threat to the image of their group and isolate her. Once conditions have reached this stage, there isn't much you as a dentist can do. One of two things will happen: either you will find her so disruptive to the team morale and efficiency that you will discharge her, or the sanctions of the group will become so strong that the individual will leave on her own accord. Either way, you are faced with the costly procedure of replacing the team member.

After reading this book, you should be struck with the interdependence of all the personnel functions. Failure to successfully execute any one of your functions as the team manager will have an impact on the group effectiveness and on the other personnel functions. If you have taken due care in the recruiting of your auxiliaries, you will be concerned with whether or not a new auxiliary will be acceptable to the team. Your chances of avoiding the disruptive influence of a deviant team member will be enhanced if you have insured that the new member has met the present team and made a favorable impression on them before you hire her. Cohesiveness will be increased if you choose auxiliaries with similar backgrounds, values, and education.

In summary, group cohesiveness can be a major attribute or a major detriment to the effectiveness of your team practice, depending upon the norms that the group forms. If the group has formed norms that are congruent with the goal of your practice, you will have an effective organization. If they are negative norms, the practice will not be effective. It is important to remember that the group will probably have more influence on the behavior of its members than you as the leader will have. Once again, group cohesiveness does not mean high productivity. High group cohesiveness means that the group will enforce its norms even if they are counter to yours.

Conflict Management

Too often the dentist tends to ignore the interpersonal problems that arise within his staff. Group effectiveness can only be attained by dealing with these problems. The conflict resolution literature lists several ways that managers tend to approach conflict within the group. One of the most common, and least effective, approaches to resolving group conflict is the tendency to ignore the fact that the conflict exists. You will have a tendency to do this because you will be uncertain about how to handle the conflict and perhaps feel that conflict within your office reflects poorly on the quality of your leadership. Therefore, you will tend to look the other way and pretend that it does not exist.

Another equally ineffective approach to conflict resolution is to encourage the members to settle their differences among themselves. When you do this, you are assuming that the conflict is based on substantive issues and not on personality differences. You are further assuming that the staff members have the necessary incentive to want to resolve their problems. Experience has shown that when the conflict is based on emotional issues, there is very little chance that the members will have the ability to successfully resolve their conflict.

Other ineffective methods are *smoothing* and *repressing.* Smoothing occurs when you use rewards such as bonuses for more effective group performance to encourage the members to settle their conflict. Repressing occurs when you use threats to force them to control their conflict so that it does not disrupt the team. Repressing generally evidences itself in comments such as "either get along together, or I'll fire you!"

Another poor technique in conflict resolution is to attempt to settle the conflict by a vote. This is normally ineffective because it intensifies a win-lose situation, which lowers commitment and satisfaction with the decision. When you vote (unless it should be unanimous), someone will win and someone will lose. Research indicates that those who lose will harbor resentment and will either actively resist the implementation of the decision, or will become passive and uncommitted.

Another solution to conflict resolution is to fire the key figures in the conflict, which can be equally ineffective since there is a high probability that they will become martyrs in the eyes of those group members who remain. Further, the people that you dismiss represent the loss of a valuable investment in trained personnel. You must now go through a period of lower productivity until you can replace these team members.

Obviously, the best solution to the resolution of conflict is to prevent it in the first place. You can do much to prevent the rise of conflict in your team by establishing clear operational goals which emphasize group performance rather than individual effectiveness. The establishment of these clear operational goals will avoid confusion and overlapping of responsibilities which can lead to conflict. Clarification of goals and the procedures designed to attain them can be greatly facilitated by the use of an office manual.

If, despite your best efforts, conflict does arise within your team, it has been found that the best approach is an open and frank discussion of differences as soon as they are detected and before emotions can become overly involved and a win-lose situation develops. You must recognize that the conflict is inevitable, and that conflict is not bad if it is handled effectively. Some conflicts are bound to occur in your team. Most of these in a well-led team will revolve around the means of attaining the organizational goals. If such conflict does not arise, it may be that your people are so disinterested in the operation that they are not committed enough to spend the energy required in a conflict. Conflict is bad when it is over emotional issues.

We have talked about how to resolve conflicts, but we also must know how to detect the signs of conflict. We will discuss some of the leading indicators of intragroup conflict. Most communications difficulties are the result of interpersonal conflict of which the group members themselves are unaware. It is seldom that when group members say they have a communications problem that communications are the primary cause. The emotions aroused by interpersonal conflict act as barriers to, or distorters of, the messages that pass between the members involved in the conflict. The members tend to filter and distort the messages and to make hostile interpretations of the intent of the messages.

As the interpersonal conflict continues, the participants tend to lose interest in their work because of the unpleasant atmosphere. This lack of interest manifests itself in chronic absenteeism or lateness plus a general feeling of malaise. The stress of the interpersonal conflicts leads to fatigue which in turn leads to a general lack of motivation and the loss of the desire to help others when required. As the dentist and leader of the group, it is your responsibility to detect these signs of interpersonal conflict and take the necessary steps to either resolve the conflict or limit its effects.

Summary

Knowledge of small group dynamics is necessary to be an effective dentist/manager. You must understand the individual differences in the needs which attract your staff to your practice and be able to meet those needs in order to motivate them. You must develop a cohesive group with desirable norms of behavior and be alert to and cope with interpersonal conflict.

Review Questions

1. Explain how group cohesiveness and group norms can interact to affect practice productivity.
2. Describe the symptoms of interpersonal conflict.
3. Discuss the possible effects of using a vote to settle a conflict.
4. Explain the differences between pivotal and peripheral norms.

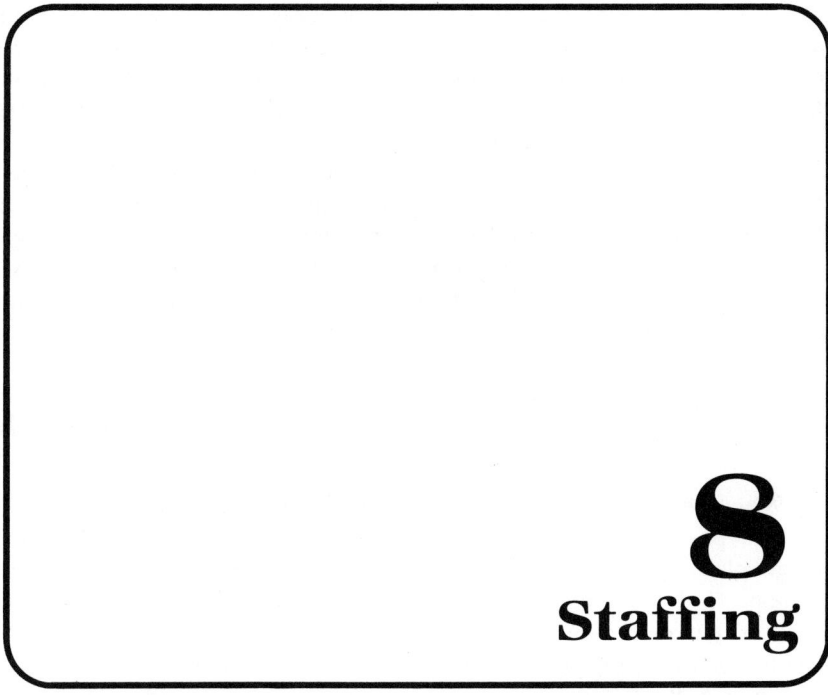

8
Staffing

Learning Objectives

Upon completion of this chapter, you should be able to:

- Develop a job description and a job specification for a dental staff member.
- Understand the biases that may affect the success of your staffing efforts.
- Comply with anti-discrimination legislation as it applies to staffing.
- Conduct an effective hiring interview.

Introduction

The purpose of the management function known as staffing is to plan for and obtain the personnel necessary to help you deliver effective dental care to your patients. This is probably the most important of all your managerial functions and yet one which is the least understood by most managers. The consequences of poor staffing are serious because they result in poor productivity, low morale, and high turnover. Consultants estimate that the cost of turnover in a dental office ranges from $7,500 to $10,000 per staff member.

This estimate includes that the cost of placing the ads and the time the dentist and his staff must take away from patient treatment to interview the applicants. It does not take into account the lowered productivity, patient alienation and the stress placed upon the dentist and his staff when they have hired an unsuitable employee. Nor does it take into account the training costs involved in hiring a replacement.

Job Description

When dentists are asked, "What is the first step in hiring staff members for your practice?", they normally respond, "Place an ad." The first step is not to place an ad, but to determine just what you want the new staff member to do. A careful review of the present duties of your staff may well indicate overlapping and duplication of duties. The way to identify this situation is to write specific job descriptions for each of your staff. Examination of well-written and accurate job descriptions should reveal any possibility of overlap and duplication.

Let's take a look at how we might develop a job description for a dental assistant, keeping in mind that the job description will vary depending upon the state laws governing the duties that may be delegated to dental assistants. We will list the various duties we want that assistant to do as follows:

- greet patient
- seat patient
- drape patient
- administer topical anesthesia
- install rubber dam
- pass instruments
- apply dycal and copalite
- collect patient data

The list could go on for some time, depending on the amount of delegation you feel comfortable with and what the state laws will permit.

Job Specifications

Now that you have a list of what you want your assistant to do, you must determine what kind of person it takes to accomplish those tasks. The first thought that probably comes to mind is to state some experience or educational requirement. While this can certainly be important, it is probably not the most important thing that you will want to look for. There are three broad areas that are of interest — personality, motivation, and knowledge/job experience. If knowledge or job experience were the sole area of interest, we could simply ask a computer to sort through the applications and choose the most experienced and/or the best educated applicant. Yet I know of no one who would hire on this basis without having seen and talked to the applicants.

You must think about what kinds of motivation you are looking for. Most will agree that you want someone who likes people and is motivated to help them. You also want someone who does not have great needs to be a leader, since you are the team leader and dental assisting requires someone who likes to work as a member of the team. Plus, you are looking for a person who believes in the importance of good health in general and dental health in particular.

There will be as many different personality requirements as there are dentists because, within limits, this is the most important of the four areas. The autocratic dentist will want an authoritarian staff member who thrives on taking orders and who will seldom take the initiative, while the dentist who likes to delegate to the maximum will want a self-confident, more aggressive type of personality who likes to work on her own. In almost all cases, it is also important to find a person who is outgoing, poised, and cheerful, who can develop a high degree of rapport with your patients.

The knowledge/experience area often provides many tradeoffs. Those who are experienced, certified dental assistants will expect a higher salary than will the inexperienced high school graduate. It is up to you to decide on the tradeoff between experience/job knowledge and cost. Remember that the experienced applicant will probably reach a high level of productivity rather rapidly, while you must expect a fairly long period of relatively low productivity while you take the time and effort to train the inexperienced dental assistant. In the end, you seldom get something for nothing.

We have now developed a list of attributes describing the type of person we are looking for. This list is known as the *job specification.* The job description defines the duties of the new staff member, and the job specification describes the kind of person it takes to do the job well.

Creating a Pool of Applicants

Our next task is to create a pool of applicants from which to choose. It is important that you develop a pool of at least 10 to 15 applicants to insure that you have a probability of finding an applicant who comes close to meeting your job specifications. It is obvious that if you have only one applicant, you have no choice and must take what is available.

There are several sources of applicants, depending upon your specifications and the size of the labor pool in your area. For example, there is normally a surplus of dental assistants around the large cities and the dental schools, and a scarcity in small towns. The two most common recruiting sources are word-of-mouth and advertising. The dental supply salesman is a good example of a word-of-mouth source. Another source of well-trained but inexperienced dental assistants and hygienists who may be personally recruited are the community colleges which offer training programs for dental assistants and hygienists. My experience has shown that employment agencies are generally a poor source.

If you decide to place an ad, you would be well advised to carefully consider the size of the ad, the wording, and the most effective days on which to run the ad. The size of the ad must be large enough to draw the attention of possible applicants. There are two important requirements for the wording of the ad. The first consideration is how much information to put in the ad, and here opinion differs. Some recommend that the ad be very specific in describing the qualifications, hours, and wages, the logic being to eliminate those who are obviously not suitable. This is probably a good approach when there is an excess of applicants, but in areas where a scarcity of applicants exists, it may only prolong the process as you may have to alter both your wages and your job specifications to fill the position.

The Selection Process

The second consideration in wording your ad is whether or not to include the telephone number of the office. Some recommend including the phone number. This has merit if you decide to have your receptionist run a telephone screening to weed out obviously unqualified applicants. In this case, it is advisable to develop a telephone checklist for her to use while conducting the telephone screening interview. You might want to include the following items:

- Name
- Address
- Phone
- Education
- Experience
- Available for work
- Can meet the office hours
- Last job held
- Job references
- Quality of voice
- Grammar

Using this screening method, a large number of applicants can be screened at a cost of approximately five minutes per applicant. For those who are acceptable, the next step is to mail them a job application.

Avoiding discrimination

Before we go further, we should address the problem of job discrimination. Federal law states that employment decisions cannot be made on the basis of sex, race, color, age, religion, origin, or handicap. In addition, each state may have additional anti-discrimination legislation, and you would be well advised to contact the human rights commission of your state to obtain a copy of their legislation.

The use of many formerly common terms are now not only considered discriminatory, but are not professional — for example "girl friday," "girl," "cleaning lady," and "credit girl." Your ad should not specify a particular age, sex, color, or nationality. You should state the nature of the task to be performed plus such other items as the working hours, and experience required. Similarly, the questionnaire used in the telephone checklist, the job application, and the interview must not include discriminatory questions.

The following are samples of discriminatory questions:

- Race
- Sex
- Age or date of birth

- Marital status
- Number of children
- Who will take care of the children
- Religious affiliation
- Husband's/wife's occupation
- Have you ever been arrested

To illustrate the attitude of some job applicants towards this line of questioning, I am quoting an article that appeared in the consumer affairs column of a Southeastern newspaper.

> "There are several questions I have been asked repeatedly as I have applied for jobs recently. These questions not only enrage me, but I feel that they insult me, and disregard my competency and enthusiasm. My husband, who was recently hired in management, was never asked any of these questions. One of these questions was a very personal one. The others were: What about your children? What will you do with them? What if they became ill?; What if you're making more money than your husband? Will he be jealous? Isn't it against the law for an interviewer to ask such questions of me? What can I do about this?"

The response was vague, but was the one usually given to such queries — that no question in itself is discriminatory, but only if it is used to discriminate in a particular situation. For example, to ask about taking care of children is all right, providing both sexes are asked that question, and the answer is not the basis for making a hiring decision. If the case were brought to court, it would seem to be rather difficult to explain why you asked the question if you were not going to use it as part of your employment decision. Further, the ethical question is not about children but is about whether or not the applicant meets your job specifications, which should be based on the true requirements of the job.

You are also technically at fault if after advertising for applicants who must meet certain specifications, you decide to hire the wife of a friend who does not meet those qualifications. Technically, you should re-advertise using the reduced criteria.

All these rules and regulations are designed to prevent discrimination, not to deny you the right to specify the kind of person you really need to do the job. Recognizing that some jobs have unique requirements, the laws provide for a means of using these specifications when it can be proven that they are necessary for job performance. For example, a producer may specify the age and sex of an applicant suitable to fill a certain role in a play. Similarly, it is legal to specify that the head of a local Catholic parish be a Catholic. It probably can also be proven that it is necessary that a hygienist present an image of good oral hygiene if she is to be able to motivate her patients on the importance of practicing good oral hygiene. The technical name for these special requirements is a *Bona Fide Occupational Qualification* and is commonly referred to as a BFOQ.

Application forms

Now that we have accomplished a preliminary screening of the applicants with the telephone checklist, we recommend that you send application forms to those who have passed the initial screening. Some dentists prefer to skip this step, but it can provide you with valuable information to aid in the selection decision. Application forms are available for purchase from many sources, or you can devise your own.

As in the case of placing the ad, purchasing application forms does not relieve you of the responsibility of complying with the anti-discrimination legislation. You must read the small print in the application form. For example, this is an excerpt from the small print on a typical application form:

> This Application For Employment and Applicant Data Record is sold for general use throughout the United States. Company assumes no responsibility for inclusion in said form of any questions which, when asked by the Employer of the Job Applicant, may violate State and/or Federal Law.

How the applicant fills out the form can give us some insight into her fitness for the position. If the form is filled out in pencil when the instructions state that the form is to be filled out in ink, and if the applicant places check marks where Xs are requested, it may indicate that the applicant pays little attention to details. If the form is sloppy with many erasures, it may indicate a real lack of motivation in applying for the position, or that the applicant is generally sloppy.

In the job experience portion of the form, look for gaps in employment which are not accounted for, which may indicate that the applicant does not wish you to know about unsatisfactory job performance during that period. Observe the frequency with which she has changed jobs, which may be an indication of a lack of motivation and follow-through. Also, compare the starting and ending salaries in each of the jobs for an indication of job progression. I also recommend that you ask for a one-paragraph explanation of why the applicant wants the job. This will give you an indication of the applicant's ability to organize her thoughts and express herself in writing.

Preparing for the interview

The next step, now that we have narrowed the field of applicants through the telephone interview and still further screening by examining the returned job applications, is to arrange to interview those who have passed the screening. Be forewarned that this is a time-consuming task and that you must arrange your schedule to permit you to give your undivided attention to these interviews. If you try to dash into the interviews between patients, you will not achieve the desired results; you will only waste time.

It is important that you prepare for the interviews, especially if you are a new dentist without an office manual. You must be prepared to answer a lot of questions posed by the job applicant. The really well-qualified applicants are not likely to be as passive as those you may have dealt with previously who, for example, were too embarrassed to ask about the wages and didn't know until their first paycheck how much they were going to earn. The new dental staff members, particularly those who have attended the community colleges or other formal training schools, have been taught how to respond to the interview and to insure that they know what the job is going to entail. Among the questions you can expect to be asked are:

- Do you require uniforms? If so, will you pay for them?
- Will you pay my dental association dues?
- How many sick days are authorized? How many days of annual leave?
- Will you pay for continuing education?

Hygienists will ask:

- How many patients will you expect me to see in a day?
- Will you expect me to do any assisting?
- Do you pay a salary, a commission, or a combination?

If you have a well-organized and well-managed office, the answers to all these questions will be in your office manual. If not, you will either have to think through these questions before the interviews or shoot from the hip in attempting to field the questions.

It is also important that you provide some means of insuring that the applicant you select fully understands the answers to those questions. If the answers are in your office manual, you can require the applicant to read and discuss the manual with you or your designated staff member prior to the final hiring decision. If you do not have the answers in your office manual, we strongly recommend that you put the answers to these questions in writing, that both you and the new employee sign the agreement, and that each of you keep a copy. We recommend this not because we expect you to go to court over some disagreement with your staff member, but because it is a good way to prevent misunderstandings. Should there be a question on the job requirements and fringe benefits, all that will be required is to refer to your copies of the agreement for clarification.

It is also important to explain exactly what the job entails during the course of the interview. It is especially important to describe any unusual or unpleasant features of the job to prevent possible future employee disillusionment which could lead to termination.

For example, there was quite a stir in the newspapers several years ago in which secretaries were complaining that serving coffee to their bosses was demeaning. I personally have never used secretaries for such things; however, the point is that if you want your employee to serve coffee as part of the job, and if you make the requirement perfectly clear at the interview and the applicant accepts the job, then there should be no surprise or indignation on the part of the employee when asked to serve coffee. The moral here is to make sure that you and your future employee know exactly what is expected before the applicant is hired.

Review of recruiting steps

The steps we have taken to this point in the staffing process are:

1. Developed a job description.
2. Developed job specifications.
3. Determined possible sources for applicants.
4. Placed an ad.
5. Accomplished a telephone pre-screening of applicants.
6. Mailed job applications to those who passed the telephone screening and used the returned applications to further reduce the field of applicants.
7. Developed an office manual, or by other means determined the answers to the many questions we expect the applicant to ask.
8. Arranged the office schedule to allow sufficient time to conduct thorough interviews with the applicants.

In all the above steps, we were careful to comply with the anti-discrimination legislation.

The interview

We still have one more step before we are ready to conduct the actual interviews. That step is to prepare the questions we intend to ask in the interview. There are actually two main techniques for conducting interviews. There is the *unstructured* interview, in which the interviewee is encouraged to talk about herself through the use of probes. The information derived from this type of interview depends upon the interviewee and is very effective in psychological counseling for the information covered. The other type of interview is known as the *structured* interview. This interview is carefully structured and standardized to insure that the same information is obtained from each of the interviewees. Research indicates that the best method for making hiring decisions is the structured interview, because it insures that information critical to the hiring decision is asked of each applicant. This will also aid in preventing discrimination, since standardized questions will be asked regardless of age, sex, race, etc.

Another important point is that the interviewer must take notes during the interview. Some consultants have advised against this, feeling that note-taking would be threatening to the applicant and thus distort the interviewer's impressions of the applicant. I feel, as do most consultants, that if note-taking is done properly, it will not detract from the effectiveness of the interview.

The note-taking should be done consistently and unobtrusively throughout the interview by keeping a pad in your lap so that the interviewee cannot see what you are writing and by taking frequent notes so that the interviewee becomes accustomed to the note-taking. This note-taking is important to the effectiveness of the interview, since research indicates that interviewers remember less than 50 percent of the information when questioned immediately after the interview. If you fail to keep notes during the interview, it is almost certain that after the first few interviews, you will not be able to differentiate among the applicants that you have interviewed.

Keeping in mind that the purpose of this whole process is to enable you to predict the job behavior of the applicant, what questions shall we ask? The questions we ask should be designed to get the applicant to talk about herself so that we can gain information on which to base the hiring decision. The best type of question for this purpose is the *open-ended* question.

The open-ended question differs from the closed-ended question in that it generally starts with who, what, where, when, and why and cannot be answered with a simple yes or no. A closed-ended question might be "Did you like your last job?" to which the applicant can respond with a yes or no, which does not really tell you much about that person. On the other hand, asking her what things she liked and disliked about the last job and why should provide a great deal of important information on her motivations.

We can simplify the structure of the interview by dividing the information we desire as indicated by the job specification into categories. For example, we mentioned three categories: personality, motivation, and knowledge/experience. There are other categories such as general appearance, speech, and education. We will use the first categorization for our examples. Under the category of personality, we might ask such questions as: "How would you describe yourself as a person?", or a more indirect question "Describe the ideal dental office." Motivation may be examined by such questions as "Describe the goals you have set for yourself in the next five years" or "Tell me the things you like to do in your job." For the knowledge/experience area you might ask questions such as "Explain the difference in the way you would teach oral hygiene to a teenager and the way you would teach it to a fifty-year-old."

It is very important to develop your list of questions before you interview. It takes too much energy and thought to try to think of the questions during the interview. You cannot devote your full attention to the applicant if you are trying to figure out what you are going to say next.

It is important to keep the applicant talking since she is your source of information. There are a number of techniques for encouraging her to talk. Make it clear in the beginning that it is her responsibility to sell herself to you and that you want to get to know her as well as possible in the time available. It often helps to start the interview with a question such as "Tell me about yourself." Applicants can also normally be encouraged to talk by nods and small gestures indicating your interest in, and approval of, what they are saying. Equally effective is the practice of paraphrasing or repeating their statements back to them and encouraging them to expand on their comments.

Biases which may affect your hiring decision

No matter how well you prepare for the interview, you will not be effective until you become aware of the factors which can distort your judgment of the candidates for selection. For our purposes, we can lump these factors together under the term *biases*. There are six biases which can distort your judgment during the interview process and perhaps cause you to select the wrong candidate. These biases are first impression, similarity, stereotype, halo, contrast, and pressure to hire.

Research has found that interviewers have a tendency to make their hiring decision in the first four minutes of the interview and spend the remainder of the interview gathering data to confirm their decision. One researcher illustrated the point by splitting a group of interviewers into two sections and exposing them to two different videotapes of simulated interviews. The same applicant dressed exactly the same, and answering the same questions in exactly the same way, was given a cup of coffee at the beginning of the interview in both tapes. In the first tape, the applicant spilled the coffee on the interviewer's desk at the beginning of the interview and in the second tape, the applicant spilled the coffee on the desk at the end of the interview. The interviewers consistently rated the applicant in the first tape lower than the same applicant in the second tape. While we have not listed it as a bias, research has also shown that negative information has far more effect on the outcome of the interview than does positive information.

It has also been shown that interviewers tend to select applicants whom the interviewers believe are similar to themselves in background and values regardless of relevance to their ability to do the job. In an experiment similar to the one previously described, the applicant described herself in the first videotape in ways that indicated that she was a typical member of the upper middle class, matching the background and values of the interviewers.

In the second videotape, she said that she was one of twelve children, whose father was a truck driver, and gave other information indicating that she was a member of the lower middle class. Again, the group receiving the upper middle class information rated the applicant higher than did the group who were given information indicating that she was from the lower middle class.

We also know that people have stereotypes of what different kinds of professions should look like, for example, the cowboy, the statesman, and the truck driver. Similarly, it has been found that interviewers have their own private image of what the ideal applicant for a certain position should look and act like although the characteristics of the stereotype seldom have anything to do with the applicant's ability to perform the job.

Halo is described by psychologists as the exaggeration of the homogeneity of the individual's characteristics or traits. This is well demonstrated by the tendency of the public to assume that a celebrity is competent in all fields. Thus we have Dr. Spock, the expert in the field of child raising, expounding in the media about international affairs. In the everyday sense, we tend to assume that attractive people are clever, intelligent, have a good personality, and will be successful in whatever task they choose.

Contrast is the tendency to compare the current candidate with those who have been previously interviewed. If the applicants previously interviewed were far above average and the present applicant is average, you will have a tendency to rate the present applicant below average. Still worse from your standpoint, if the previous applicants have been far below average, the current average applicant will really shine by comparison and you will have to use considerable self-control to resist the urge to hire her on the spot.

The last bias is pressure to hire. When a staff member quits unexpectedly, all the other members of the staff, including you, must work harder to carry the work load. As the patient backlog builds up and the stress of trying to keep to the schedule becomes greater, there will be a tendency to cut short the entire staffing process and grab the first applicant you can find, with often disastrous results — the applicant proves to be unsatisfactory and you must then start the staffing process all over again.

We suggest that you avoid this situation by locating a source of temporary help while you are conducting the staffing process. In the smaller towns, it is fairly easy to develop a list of names of former assistants, hygienists, and other dental staff members who have withdrawn from dental practice to raise a family or for other reasons. These experienced people are often available for temporary hire. In the larger cities, there are organizations similar to the *Kelly Girls* who will furnish experienced dental staff members on a temporary or part-time basis.

Before you make your final hiring decision, you should involve the members of your staff in that decision by having them meet with the final two or three applicants without you being present. There are three good reasons for this. One, the candidates tend to drop their guard when they are with the employees and show more of their true nature. There is quite a bit of difference between the applicant who only asks about the fringe benefits and the one who asks questions about how the dentist feels about preventive dentistry and how well he treats the patient. The second applicant is far more likely to be motivated toward being a good staff member.

Second, the employees tend to be very observant when asked to look over a potential employee. Thus they can often add much useful information upon which to base the final decision. Third, when the staff members recommend hiring a candidate, they are making a public commitment to seeing that the new employee is a success — otherwise they will have to admit, if only to themselves, that they have made a bad decision.

This procedure can also save you valuable time if you can schedule the interviewee to see the staff prior to the interview. During this visit, members of your staff can discuss your fringe benefits and other materials contained in your office manual with the applicant prior to your interview, reducing the amount of time you will have to spend discussing these matters with the applicant.

An important matter not to be overlooked in the interview is that of job references as opposed to other types of references. References, other than job references, tend to add little information because the applicant is usually wise enough to submit only the names of non-job references who they know will give glowing recommendations.

Job references, on the other hand, are one of the best indicators of future performance if care is taken to check the references correctly. Normally the second-last employer is more reliable than the last employer, since time tends to reduce emotional bias and add perspective. In these days of litigation, you will find it difficult to get a true evaluation of the applicant from a former employer. Since they are reluctant to put unfavorable information in writing, the telephone is the best way to obtain the desired information. Even then it sometimes requires persistence to get the employer to talk.

Once you have the employer on the phone, you should have a prepared list of questions to ask so as not to waste his time and to make sure that you ask the right questions. Some of the types of questions you should ask include:

- absenteeism and tardiness
- initiative
- ability to get along with others
- strengths and weaknesses
- last, and most important, would you hire the applicant again if given the chance?

Another important means of protecting the practice is to bond your employees, especially those who deal with funds. During the interview, you should ask the candidate if she would mind being bonded. Those who really have something to hide may not say no to the request, but they also normally will not respond to the additional steps in the hiring procedure. Bonding is a relatively inexpensive way of sharing the risk of embezzlement or theft. At this writing, for example, the cost of bonding an employee for $30,000 amounts to $95 per year per employee.

We have now covered the steps in the staffing process except for terminating the interview. No matter what your evaluation of the candidate, you must treat each one with the utmost courtesy, not only for ethical reasons, but because it is important to maintain the best possible image with all members of the public and especially with members of the dental profession. It has been my experience that hygienists, dental assistants and receptionists discuss the dentists in their local area and know who is a good employer and who is not. Those with a reputation for being a good employer have little trouble getting applications from the best dental staff members in the field, while those with a poor reputation have trouble getting enough applicants to give themselves the freedom of choice and often must settle for second best in the job market.

Summary

Staffing is one of the most important and yet most poorly executed functions of a dental practice. Failure to properly staff your practice can be costly not only in terms of dollars but can also result in high levels of stress for you and your staff plus failure to deliver optimum dental care to your patients.

The staffing process should commence with the development of a job description and specification and the development of a pool of applicants. The procedure must permit you to choose the applicant with the highest probability of successfully performing in your practice. During this process, you have both an ethical and a legal responsibility to comply with anti-discrimination legislation.

Review Questions

1. Explain the difference between a job description and a job specification.
2. Discuss the types of biases which can adversely affect the hiring decision.
3. Describe the type of interview and the type of questions which have been found to be the most effective in the staffing process.

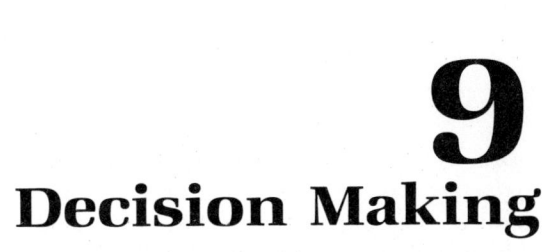

Decision Making

Learning Objectives

Upon completion of this chapter, you should be able to:

- Describe the three major considerations in the decision-making process.
- Analyze a situation using Vroom's decision-making model and select the appropriate decision-making mode.
- Recognize the pitfalls that can result from applying the wrong decision-making process.

Introduction

In the discussion of management by objectives in Chapter 1, we mentioned briefly that one of the most persistent and controversial issues in the study of management is that of participation in decision making by subordinates. You may recall that we found that research evidence provides some, but not overwhelming, support for beliefs in the efficacy of participative management. Some studies have indicated that impressive increases in productivity can be brought about by giving your subordinates an opportunity to participate in decision making. On the other hand, other researchers have found no significant differences in the productivity between subordinates who did and those who did not participate in decisions regarding the introduction of changes. Therefore, with the present evidence we must conclude, as have others, that participation in decision making has consequences that vary from one situation to another.

Vroom and Yetton's Decision-making Process

Drs. Victor H. Vroom and Phillip W. Yetton, in *Leadership and Decision-making,* have developed a procedure for determining the most effective method of decision making. They first divided the situations into group problems and individual problems. If a problem or decision clearly affects only one staff member, you would choose among the methods shown in the right-hand column of Figure 9–1. If it had potential effects on more than one staff member or on the group, you would choose among the methods shown in the left-hand column.

Both columns are arranged from top to bottom in terms of the opportunity for subordinates to influence the solution to the problem. Note that each of the alternative actions is labeled A, C, D, or G. The letters in this code signify the basic properties of the process. (A stands for the autocratic; C for the consultative; G for the group; and D for the delegated method of decision making.) The Roman numerals that follow letters constitute variations on that process. Thus, AI represents the first variation on the autocratic method, AII the second variant, and so on.

As we have said, no one decision-making method is applicable to all situations; the function of this model should be to provide a framework for analysis of the situational requirements that can be translated into a prescription for decision making in a particular situation. This method of decision making is based upon an analysis of the particular problem to be solved and the context in which the problem occurs. We want to emphasize that the method used in response to one situation should not constrain the method or style used in other situations.

Group problems	Individual problems
AI. You solve the problem or make the decision yourself, using information available to you at the time.	AI. You solve the problem or make the decision by yourself, using information available to you at the time.
AII. You obtain the necessary information from your subordinates, then decide the solution to the problem yourself. You may or may not tell your subordinates what the problem is in getting the information from them. The role played by your subordinates in making the decision is clearly one of providing the necessary information to you, rather than generating or evaluating alternative solutions.	AII. You obtain the necessary information from your subordinate, then decide on the solution to the problem yourself. You may or may not tell the subordinate what the problem is in getting the information from him. His role in making the decision is clearly one of providing the necessary information to you, rather than generating or evaluating alternative solutions.
CI. You share the problem with the relevant subordinates individually, getting their ideas and suggestions without bringing them together as a group. Then *you* make the decision, which may or may not reflect your subordinates' influence.	CI. You share the problem with your subordinate, getting his ideas and suggestions. Then you make a decision, which may or may not reflect his influence.
CII. You share the problem with your subordinates as a group, obtaining their collective ideas and suggestions. Then you make the decision, which may or may not reflect your subordinates' influence.	GI. You share the problem with your subordinate, and together you analyze the problem and arrive at a mutually agreeable solution.
GII. You share the problem with your subordinates as a group. Together you generate and evaluate alternatives and attempt to reach agreement (consensus) on a solution. Your role is much like that of chairman. You do not try to influence the group to adopt "your" solution, and you are willing to accept and implement any solution which has the support of the entire group.	DI. You delegate the problem to your subordinate, providing him with any relevant information that you possess, but giving him responsibility for solving the problem by himself. You may or may not request him to tell you what solution he has reached.

Figure 9–1 Decision methods for group and individual problems. (Reprinted from *Leadership and Decision-making* by Victor H. Vroom and Phillip W. Yetton by permission of the University of Pittsburgh Press. © 1973 by the University of Pittsburgh Press.)

The three major considerations

There are three major considerations that distinguish the effectiveness of the decision-making process. These are:

1. the *quality* or rationality of the decision;
2. the *acceptance* of the decision by subordinates and their commitment to execute it effectively; and
3. the amount of *time* required to make the decision.

It would be naive to think that group decision making is always more effective than autocratic decision making or vice versa. The relative effectiveness of these two extreme methods depends upon the importance attached to quality, acceptance and time variables in the solution to a particular decision.

You will face some problems wherein you will feel indifferent toward the possible solutions since one answer is as good as another from your standpoint, provided that those who have to carry them out are committed to them. For example, it shouldn't matter to you when each member of your staff takes her vacation, provided they comply with certain constraints that you may provide, such as that you will always have adequate clinical coverage in each specialty. There are, however, decisions in which the quality of the decision is all-important, such as the financing arrangement for your practice, whether or not you will lease or purchase your equipment, etc.

The next consideration concerns the importance of the acceptance of the decision. Here you are concerned with the preferences of your subordinates and their feelings about the alternative solutions to the problem, or the extent to which acceptance or commitment on the part of your subordinates is critical to the effective implementation of the decision.

In most situations, the effectiveness of an organizational decision is influenced both by its quality or rationality and by the extent to which it is accepted by your subordinates. In these cases, your decision can be ineffective for two reasons: (1) because you did not utilize all the available information resulting in a poor decision, or (2) you made a decision which was resisted and opposed by those members of your staff who had to implement it.

There will be some cases in which your subordinates are not involved in the execution of the decision. This may well be the case in the decision we discussed a moment ago in which you were deciding whether to lease or purchase your equipment. In decisions such as this, you are the sole implementer of the decision and it is unlikely that acceptance by your subordinates would be required. In the second type of situation in which acceptance or commitment to the decision by subordinates is critical, you have still another factor to consider. There will be some cases in which acceptance or commitment to the decision by your subordinates is not critical because you are able to monitor or observe their actions and to control their rewards and punishments.

In most organizations, people are sometimes required to carry out decisions to which they feel no personal commitment, or even to which they are strongly opposed. If you are faced with this situation, you must consider whether the actions of your staff will be observable by you so that you can make sure the decisions are carried out. This requires that you control the reward and/or penalties which are meted out in accordance with the degree of compliance desired.

With the close interaction required in a dental setting, you are most often in a position to very closely monitor the performance and actions of your staff. Acceptance becomes more critical as the effective execution of the decision requires initiative, judgment, or commitment and when you cannot directly observe the auxiliary's performance. For example, the receptionist interacts frequently with the patients in ways which you cannot directly observe such as telephone conversations, bill collecting, and making appointments. Similarly, there are periods when the dental assistant or hygienist is alone with the patient, and you must rely on her commitment to the practice and its objectives rather than on your direct observations and control.

Another important factor in the decision-making process is the consideration of the time available versus the time required to reach a decision. Remember that group decision making is the most time-consuming and, therefore, the most expensive. Let us take a hypothetical situation to illustrate the point. Assume that you and your staff, consisting of one auxiliary and one receptionist, both earning $9,000 a year, become involved in solving a problem and arriving at a decision which takes one hour on the part of the three of you. Let's further assume that you are netting $20,000 a year as your own salary. Therefore, your auxiliary and receptionist are each being paid approximately $5.00 an hour for their time, and you are being paid $11.00 an hour. Let's further consider the alternative use of your time from the standpoint of your income. The average unassisted dentist approximates a gross of $60.00 per hour. If you have spent an hour with your auxiliary and receptionist attempting to arrive at the solution to a problem, the price of that decision is $10.00 an hour for the use of the auxiliary and the receptionist, plus $11.00 an hour for the use of your time, plus a loss of income of $60.00 that could have been gained from treating patients, for a total cost of $81.00. There are certainly many decisions which are so important that $81.00 an hour is not an unreasonable cost to assure the quality of the decision. You will also face many decisions which are not worth the expense involved in using the group decision-making process.

We have now seen that there are three major factors that affect the decision-making process: (1) the quality of the decision; (2) the acceptance of the decision; and (3) the time required or available to make the decision.

Applying the model

Now take a look at the decision-making model in Figure 9-2. As we go through a few examples of how to apply the steps in the decision-making model, I hope you will be struck by the fact that there is no one best way, or any guarantee of success, in any decision-making procedure thus far invented. As you go through the solutions to these problems, I also hope you will be impressed by the fact that the key to effective decision making is your ability to assess the factors in the situation. This model is an effective aid to the decision-making process but it cannot replace good judgment.

Assume that you are faced with a decision about whether to buy or lease some additional equipment you feel you need for your practice. Looking at the chart in Figure 9-2 under A, you are asked "Is there a quality requirement such that one solution is likely to be more rational than another?" This step will assist you in protecting the quality of your decision. In this case, your decision can have important ramifications for the future of the practice; therefore, you must insure a high-quality decision.

Following the Yes line from A, the next question is "Do I have sufficient information to make a high-quality decision?" The answer is most likely to be Yes. If the answer were No, you would have to consider if your staff might have the information, and if so to consult them by following the path marked No. (Notice that in this case, the end solutions delete the AI, AII alternatives since you would be unable to make a high-quality decision by yourself because you lack the necessary information.)

Following the Yes line leads you to D, "Is acceptance of decision by subordinates critical to effective implementation?" In this case, since you are the only one whose actions are required to implement the decision, the answer will be No.

Following the No line from question D, you skip question E because it is irrelevant, which leads you to F, "Do subordinates share the organizational goals . . . ?" Observe that the only difference between the final two

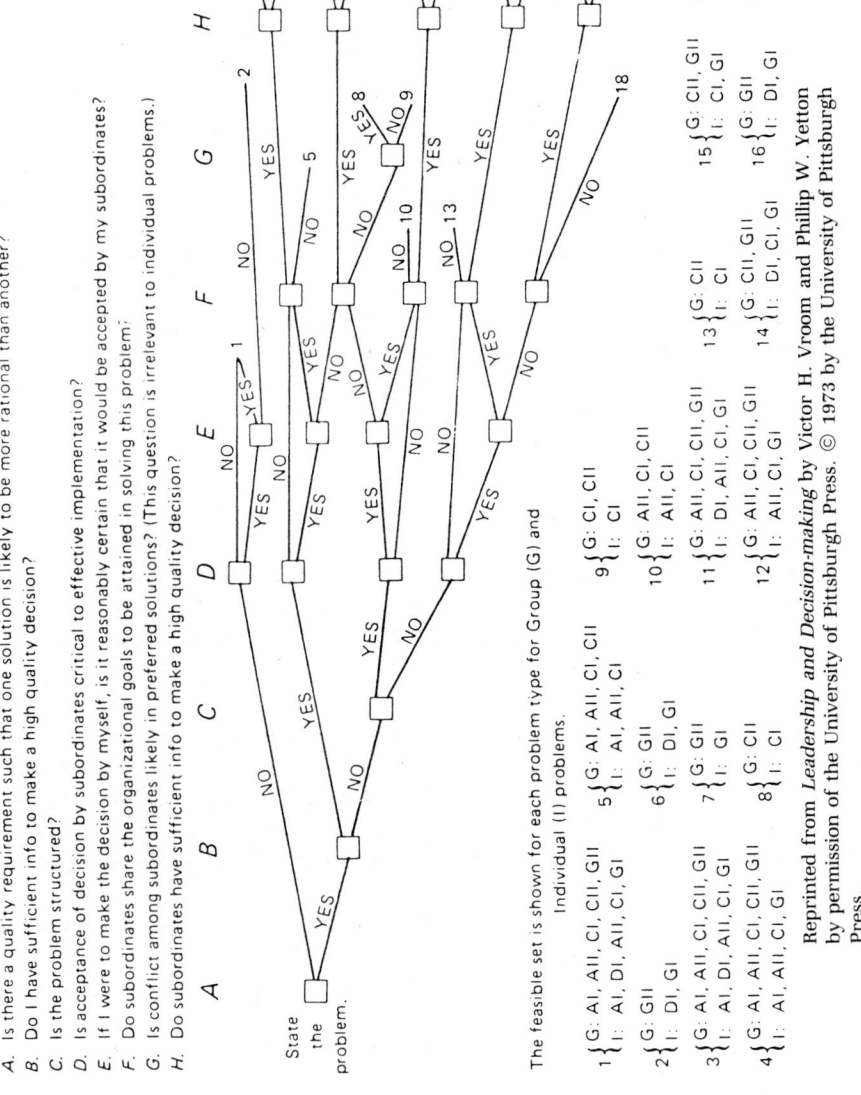

Figure 9-2 Decision-process flow chart for both individual and group problems

alternatives from here is that if you feel that your staff shares the organizational goals, you have GII (sharing the problem with your subordinates as a group . . .) as an alternative, while if they do not share the goals of the practice, you do not have that option. The rationale is that if your staff does not share the organizational goals, group problem solving is not an effective way to make decisions.

Typical cases in which dental staffs do not share the practice goals occur when the staff is professionally immature and can only see the importance of their own portion of the practice. Here the hygienist feels that the practice should revolve around her recall system and that everything else is secondary, while the receptionist feels that running a neat, efficient office is the key to practice success and that all other considerations should revolve around her activities.

You can see that when your staff has this type of outlook, there is little chance of utilizing a group problem-solving approach effectively.

One possible way of preventing this situation where possible is to rotate the duties of your staff members occasionally. For example, having your hygienist work as a chairside assistant or assisting the receptionist on occasion is a good way to broaden her perspective.

To summarize, in this particular example, you were faced with a situation where a high-quality decision was necessary, you had sufficient information available, and staff members were not required to implement the decision so that acceptance was not a consideration. This left you with a choice of all the alternatives from AI to GII if the staff shares your practice goals (or deleting the group decision-making alternative GII if they do not share your practice goals).

Now take a problem such as determining the vacation schedule for your staff. The answer to block A on the quality requirement can probably be answered No because one schedule would be as good as another as far as you are concerned, as long as the staff follows your guidance on how many members can be gone at the same time, or what members of the staff must be available at specified times.

In this case, you would follow the No line from block A, skipping blocks B and C which are now irrelevant, to block D. Your answer to block D, "Is acceptance of decision by subordinates critical to effective implementation?", may be a difficult one, requiring judgment on your part. In most cases, you can force implementation of your decision on the vacation schedule even if the staff feels that your decision was arbitrary and unfair.

However, if in addition you make the decision when the answer to block E "acceptance of the decision" is No, in some rare cases, one of your staff may fake an illness or even quit to keep her vacation schedule.

Equally important is the possibility of increased resentment and lowered morale on the part of your staff because they were forced to accept your decision. While they will carry out their duties under these conditions, the lowered morale can be unpleasant for both you and the patients who are quick to sense subtle changes in the environment.

Let's assume that you will agree with me that in most cases where quality is not a consideration and where decision will affect the staff, they should be permitted to participate, *providing* that conflict among them is not expected. I recommend adding Block G (see Figure 9–2) to the chain of decisions on decision alternatives for Problem 2 because decisions should not be referred to the staff if conflict among subordinates is likely.

Where quality is not a consideration and you are considering whether to have your staff participate, you must always consider block G. If you fail to consider the implications of block G and use GII as recommended, you may risk setting up a serious conflict situation which will only add to any rifts and dissensions in your staff.

If you have been unfortunate in selecting your staff members, and cliques or uncooperativeness have developed between staff members, I would not recommend using GII for any decisions affecting the staff. It is better to use either CI or CII, which will give the staff members an opportunity to express their opinions and desires, but which will lessen the chances for staff conflict.

To this point, we have not considered time, the third consideration in decision making. Time is money in your practice and should be conserved when possible. The alternatives in Figure 9–1 are listed from top to bottom in order of the time consumed, with the shortest time being required for the autocratic methods and the longest time for the group method. Given a set of alternatives, choosing from the recommended alternatives on the left in Figure 9–2 will result in the least expensive method from the time standpoint.

Another consideration on the same scale as the time dimension, is that of staff development. If you see no need to develop your staff to prepare them for promotion or to permit them to accept more delegation, the available alternative requiring the shortest time should be chosen. If you wish to develop your staff, then the method requiring the most participation is recommended although it is more expensive in terms of time. It is important also to make the decision about whether the short-term savings in time are more important than the long-term gains of a more professional staff.

As managers, we sometimes overestimate the amount of participation desired by our staff. It is a good idea to develop an agreement with your staff so that they can be honest and tell you when they don't desire to participate. This way time will not be wasted gaining their participation when they are willing to accept your decision.

Dentist personality and decision making

Your personality is another consideration in determining the proper method to use for decision making. If your personality tends to be authoritarian, you will be biased to evaluate situations so that they call for the AI/AII type of decision making. In this case, you must have the knowledge and information required to make the decisions yourself. If you are the type who believes in participative management, you will have a tendency to use the consultative and group methods of decision-making alternatives. In this event, you should hire staff members who desire to participate in decision making. In addition, you will have to develop skills in leading group discussions and be psychologically prepared to accept the decisions made by your staff.

Summary

Despite the claims of those who advocate the participative style of management, there does not appear to be any one best way to make decisions. The model developed by Vroom and Yetton does provide a logical framework for deciding what method to use under differing conditions.

The model is based upon protecting three key elements in the decision: the quality of the decision, acceptance of the decision by the staff, and the time cost of the decision.

Effective use of the model requires the ability to accurately assess the situation in terms of Vroom and Yetton's criteria. To do this, you must avoid personal bias and develop the skills to implement the decision-making modes, such as knowledge of the practice in the authoritarian modes, and the ability to conduct group discussions in the participative modes.

Review Questions

1. List the three major considerations in the decision-making process.
2. Employee participation in decision making is appropriate when (*choose one*):
    a. Acceptance requirements are high and quality requirements are low.
    b. Acceptance requirements are low and quality requirements are high.

3. If there is a requirement for a high-quality decision and the decision will be implemented by someone outside your dental practice, you should permit the staff to participate in the decision.
   True_____   False_____
4. Acceptance of your decisions by your dental assistant is more important than acceptance by your receptionist.
   True_____   False_____

10
Performance Appraisal in a Dental Practice

Learning Objectives

Upon completion of this chapter, you should be able to:

- List and describe the biases which may detract from the effectiveness of your performance appraisal program.
- Discuss the legal implications of a performance appraisal program.
- Discuss how your personality may affect your performance appraisal interview.
- Prepare for and conduct an effective performance appraisal program.

Introduction

In Chapter 1, we discussed the procedures for setting performance standards/goals and objectives and how to use them to control auxiliary performance. Now it is time to consider how performance appraisal fits into the control process.

Performance appraisal is exactly that, a means of appraising the performance of your staff members against the stated performance standards/goals. It is a formal discussion between you and your auxiliary to:

1. Determine how well she is performing and why.
2. Determine how she can do even better in the future so that both she and the practice can benefit.

We have previously discussed the value of feedback for informing the individual about how well she is doing in meeting the standard/goals. There are numerous forms of feedback. There is continuous feedback that goes on in your practice from day to day as you comment either casually, or more formally, to one of your staff members about how well she is doing on a particular task. This form of feedback is very important because learning theory has proven that the closer to the performance the feedback occurs, the more effective it becomes.

If you look back to your own experience in work situations where you were the subordinate, you probably received numerous feedback comments on your performance from your superiors over a period of time, some good and some bad. While you were told how well or how poorly you accomplished a particular task, you did not know how well you were doing overall. You may have been criticized on some tasks and praised on others, but you were never quite certain as to what was considered important and unimportant in your task performance. This is the reason that the formal performance appraisal is so important. The formal performance appraisal is the best means for reviewing the overall performance of your auxiliaries in a manner that clearly identifies how well they are doing.

Advantages of Performance Appraisal

An effective performance appraisal program will do many things for you. It will:

- Measure the effectiveness of your personnel selection procedures so that you will be able to tell how good your sources of personnel recruitment are. For example, if you consistently used the same source for recruitment and found that the job applicants you hired from that source were generally below average in performance, you would want to search elsewhere for new sources.

- Provide a means of evaluating the effectiveness of your training programs, since poor training is often the cause of substandard performance.
- Provide an unbiased basis for determining pay increases and suitability for promotion.
- Improve the motivation and performance of your subordinates by providing formal feedback and involving them in self-evaluation of their performance.
- Provide a well-documented, legal and ethical program for determining when termination is required for failure to meet the performance standards.

The documentation procedures involved in an effective performance appraisal program should meet the legal requirements for termination under the Equal Opportunity guidelines.

This last area is one that is rapidly increasing in importance. While the relatively small organizations such as the dental office have not yet had major problems in this area, larger organizations are finding that performance appraisal is being increasingly scrutinized by the legal system. There have been cases in other professions in which a worker has been terminated and subsequently has taken the case to court. In those cases in which the court has found for the worker, the court has required that the employer pay the worker back wages and continue to pay wages until the terminated employee found suitable employment. This situation can be avoided by maintaining a well-documented performance appraisal program.

Dentist Personality and Performance Appraisal

Now that we have taken a look at the reason for the performance appraisal, consider some of the dimensions of your behavior as a dentist that might either help or defeat the performance appraisal. All human behavior can be categorized into one of the four quadrants as shown in Figure 10-1. As you can see, the vertical dimension ranges from *dominant* behavior, characterized by a willingness to take control of the situation and to lead others. At the other end of this dominant dimension, we have *submissive* behavior, i.e., submitting to the control by others.

The horizontal line contains the friendly-hostile behavior dimension. *Hostile* behavior is a suspicious, unfriendly, uncaring approach to others

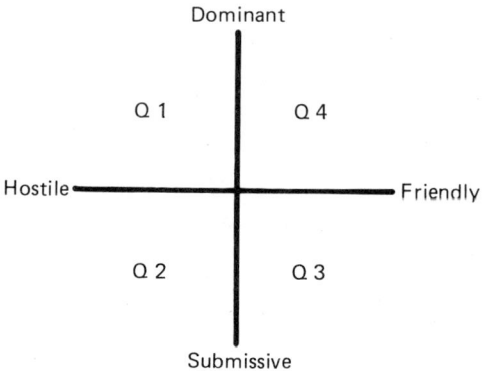

Figure 10–1 Behavioral dimensions

which has little concern or respect for the values and feelings of others. At the other end of the dimension, we have *friendly* behavior, which means a basic trust in, and a regard for, others. Friendly behavior is a frank, empathetic, and trusting approach to people.

While it is very unusual for an individual's behavior to consistently stay at one point in any of these quadrants, each individual's overall behavior may be characterized by the behavior described by one of these quadrants. For further clarification, look at an example of how one individual's behavior might vary during a particular day. If you were a professor in the College of Dentistry talking with one of the students, you might adopt the dominant/friendly behaviors of quadrant I. On the other hand, when talking to the Dean, you might move to quadrant III and be friendly and submissive.

For still another example: if you were a parent with a young child, you might call to little Johnnie using quadrant IV behavior, saying "Johnnie, please come in and wash your hands. Dinner is ready." Should Johnnie ignore you, the next call might be more insistent. You are now moving from someplace in the upper right of quadrant IV toward quadrant I. If little Johnnie still ignores your calls, you might move into the dominant-hostile quadrant I by saying "Johnnie, get in here and wash your hands or I'll spank you!" So we see that an individual's behavior may move freely among the four quadrants depending upon the situation.

However, in general most people seem to favor one quadrant over the others. A dentist who is in quadrant I (dominant-hostile) conducts a performance appraisal by acting as the judge and telling his people exactly how he feels about their performance. The conversation is all one-way, from himself to his auxiliary, with little regard for the feelings of that auxiliary or possible facts in the situation. This kind of a boss feels that the only way to keep the people performing is to keep them running scared. Tell them what to do and watch them closely to make sure they do it. If they don't do what you tell them to, fire them. This type of management will often result in high performance in the short run, but it may also lead to high turnover and low initiative on the part of the auxiliaries in the long run.

A dentist using quadrant II behavior (submissive-hostile) in a performance appraisal interview is most likely to feel that the performance appraisal is really not worthwhile. People are lackadaisical, and it won't change them much anyway, so why bother? In this case, the performance appraisal interview is routine and mechanical. Little is accomplished for future development by this type of appraisal, since the auxiliary usually comes out confused or unsure about how she is doing or how she can improve. As a result, she usually feels cheated or let down, thinking "I was really hoping for a real appraisal and all I got was a fast shuffle."

Behavior characterized by quadrant III (submissive-friendly) is probably what is most commonly observed in a performance appraisal. The quadrant III dentist has a high need for being liked and is not likely to risk any confrontation or take a chance that what he says will offend his subordinate.

The appraisal is easygoing and optimistic — when performance is just average, he exaggerates the performance level to outstanding, and when performance is below average, he is always ready to make excuses for the auxiliary. An interview of this type has two possible results. The auxiliary either leaves feeling that she is doing much better than she really is and that there is no need for improvement, or she leaves the meeting feeling that her dentist really doesn't know what is going on, and so there is no need to make any improvements in her performance.

The truly effective performance appraisal is characterized by those dentists who operate in the dominant-friendly quadrant IV. Here the appraisal is businesslike and uses a problem-solving approach whose objective is to see how *we* can do better. It involves both you and your auxiliary in a searching analysis and discussion based on solid evidence. The result is an accurate, balanced appraisal resulting in a workable plan of action for the future. Of the four approaches, this approach normally gives you the best chance of obtaining superior results.

Motivational Aspects of Performance Appraisal

The motivational paradigm can be used to better understand the motivational aspects of the performance appraisal program. The basic motivational paradigm is: $M = f(E \rightarrow P) \times (P \rightarrow O) V$. The motivation of an individual (M) is a function of that individual's perceptions of the probability that his or her effort (E) will lead to effective or improved performance (P) times the probability that if she effectively performs, it will lead to an outcome (O) times the value (V) that she places on the outcome.

The performance appraisal interview provides the feedback which tells the auxiliary whether or not her effort has truly led to satisfactory performance, and the coaching and discussion during the performance appraisal interview serve to strengthen her belief that the effort can truly lead to or approach the desired performance. The positive and constructive feedback furnished during the interview should also provide a positive outcome (O) which is valued by the auxiliary. In those cases in which performance has not been met, the feedback is negative and provides her with a negatively valued outcome. Theory has led us to believe that she will increase performance to avoid this negative feedback.

As you will see in the procedures for conducting an effective performance appraisal interview, one of the items that will be clarified is the value that the auxiliary places on the outcome (O) she has been receiving. It takes little thought to realize that outcomes valued by one person may not be valued by another. For example, most supervisors feel that pay is the outcome valued most by subordinates, while when subordinates are questioned, positive feedback often turns out to be the number one outcome valued by the subordinates.

In the end, the key question is not "are the staff's goals being met," but "are the practice goals being met?" However, if the subordinate's goals are not being met, she is very unlikely to be motivated toward meeting the performance standards and objectives of the practice.

Traditional vs. Effective Performance Appraisal

The traditional performance appraisal programs used in the past consisted primarily of a meeting between the supervisor and the subordinate entailing a one-way conversation. The supervisor detailed the successes and shortcomings of the subordinate item by item. Recent research has found such performance appraisal programs to be ineffective. The reasons for the ineffectiveness of these programs are numerous, but can be categorized into two areas: (1) the reaction of the superior, and (2) the reaction of the subordinate. The traditional performance appraisal interview most often used a judgmental approach. This was as unpleasant to the superior as it was to the subordinate; because the superior felt that he was "playing God" in making criticisms which could affect the future welfare of the subordinate, while the subordinate feared being subjected to the judgment of the supervisor.

Further, while it is easy to conduct a performance appraisal interview with either a passive or a successful employee, an interview conducted with an aggressive employee who is performing in a substandard manner involves a great deal of criticism and/or confrontation, which both the employer and subordinate find extremely unpleasant. As a result, traditional performance appraisals are normally only conducted when the superior is forced to do so by the policies of the organization.

When they are required to do these performance appraisals, the average supervisor tries to gloss over the subordinate's shortcomings, or make a short and superficial performance appraisal interview. Such an interview is normally so unstructured that, when questioned, the subordinates do not realize that they have actually been through a performance appraisal interview. When subordinates are criticized in a traditional performance appraisal interview, they tend to become defensive and performance does not increase. However, performance does increase in those areas in which they are praised, leading to the conclusion that criticism lowers the subordinate's motivation to improve performance.

As compared to the traditional approach to performance appraisal, the new approach builds on the previous steps of setting performance standards and goals which permit self-evaluation or automatic feedback to the employee. It further uses the participative problem-solving approach to the evaluation of auxiliary performance. As will be seen when we discuss the procedures for the performance appraisal interview, the problem-solving approach avoids the judgmental approach and the criticism that arouses defensiveness and lowers the motivation of staff members.

Biases and Performance Appraisal

The success of your performance appraisal program rests in large part on your ability to recognize and overcome biases that prevent you from accurately evaluating the performance of your staff members.

The first bias is *halo,* which is a tendency to let performance on one facet of a job color your evaluation of the staff member's overall job performance. For example, if one of the dental assistants is extremely successful in establishing patient rapport, it is possible that you would let this successful performance outweigh poor performance in keeping records, four-handed dentistry, and operatory preparation. She would then be getting by with a far less effective performance than she should.

Recency is a bias that occurs when you permit recent, short-term performance to overshadow your opinion of the auxiliary's long-term performance. Just as some children become angels in the few weeks before Christmas and terrors the rest of the year, so some of your staff will have a tendency to become very effective just a few weeks before the performance appraisal and then revert back to substandard after the appraisal. You should also be sympathetic to the auxiliary who has an uncharacteristically bad couple of weeks just before the appraisal and weigh it against her superior long-term performance.

Contrast is the tendency to compare performance of one dental assistant to that of other dental assistants without regard to the amount of experience, or other mitigating circumstances. This may make the more experienced staff members seem superior to the newer staff members. What you may have forgotten is that the experienced staff members' performance when they first started was no better than that of the new staff member.

Inconsistency occurs when you waver in your acceptance of different levels of performance standards/goals. One day you will accept substandard performance by labeling it satisfactory, while on other days you consider a very high level of performance only minimally satisfactory.

Preparation for the Performance Appraisal Interview

The first step in preparing for the performance appraisal interview is to measure performance on those key result areas of the job description on which you have established performance standards/goals. This requires an administrative system within your practice to furnish you and your staff with data on their performance so that it can be compared to their performance standards/goals (as was discussed in Chapter 1).

Also as discussed in Chapter 1, because of the importance of self-generated feedback in increasing auxiliary motivation, the responsibility for gathering data on their performance should be delegated to each staff member. You in turn should note typical examples of good and poor performance during the rating period as the events occur. This requires discipline on your part. Keeping 3 × 5 cards in your pocket will assist you in noting these events, after which you can drop them in the individual's file for review just before the performance appraisal.

A few weeks before the performance appraisal, you and your auxiliary should start preparation for the interview. Research indicates that the more time your auxiliary spends preparing for, and the more involved she becomes in the conduct of the interview, the greater the improvement in her post-interview performance. You can help your auxiliary to prepare by sending her a note setting the time, place and date for the performance appraisal and informing her that she will be expected to lead the evaluation by covering the following areas.

1. What performance standards/goals were met.
2. What goals/standards were not met, and her recommended action on these standards/goals.
3. What performance standards and goals should be set for the next rating program.
4. What other recommendations she may have for other areas of the practice.

The results of your first attempt to conduct this type of performance appraisal program may be disappointing, for few dental auxiliaries will have had any experience in such a program. They will have to be encouraged and coached before they can truly benefit from it. As an auxiliary becomes experienced in performance appraisal, she will do most of the talking, but in the beginning you may have to lead her a little.

In opening the interview, try to establish rapport with the auxiliary and once again explain that the purpose of the interview is to review *our* performance as a team to see how *we* can improve our efficiency and that of the practice as a whole.

You will find that this type of interview relieves you of a lot of pressure, in that the auxiliary will normally be far more critical of her performance than you and that rather than having to criticize her performance, you simply have to nod in agreement at her self-criticism.

Where she has fallen short of the performance standards, it is important to ask her what recommendations she has for improving her performance. A discussion of improvement methods now becomes a team problem-solving effort rather than a judging session. Research indicates that criticism of performance by the boss seldom improves performance, while self-discovery of shortcomings and the use of the problem-solving approach to removing performance obstacles does improve performance.

Just as nothing works perfectly, there will be occasions where the auxiliary has an exaggerated opinion of her performance and is unable to detect her own substandard performance. In this case the use of probes should lead her to self-discovery of her problems. For example, if she reports that she has done an excellent job in meeting your standards of patient rapport, you might ask her why Mrs. Murphy left in such a huff last week, and why Mr. Jones hasn't been back. Normally, careful probing can avoid the need for you to directly criticize her performance. In other cases, you will find that the auxiliary did not really attempt to meet the performance standard because she didn't understand the reason for it.

I recently sat in on a performance appraisal interview in which the auxiliary reported that she had failed to warm the anesthesia carpules as required by the performance standard. When asked what the problem was, she simply shrugged and said, "I just don't seem to be able to remember to do it." The dentist asked her to please try harder to remember and started to move on with the interview. I interrupted to ask her if she knew why she was to warm the carpule, and she said, "No." When the reason was explained, her subsequent performance met the standard because the standard was now meaningful to her. She now knew that warming the carpule might reduce the pain of the injection to the patient.

In the worst case, you will occasionally encounter the auxiliary who will stubbornly refuse to accept her shortcomings, or refuse to accept the reasons for some of the standards. In this case, unpleasant as it may be, you will have to resort to the dominant-friendly behavior and firmly explain to the auxiliary that meeting the standards is essential to the success of your practice and that failure to meet these standards within the next reporting period will result in termination of her employment.

At the end of the interview you should have in writing a revised set of performance standards/goals with the action steps necessary to achieve them, and have devised the administrative procedures necessary to measure the performance.

Common Errors in Performance Appraisal

When giving a performance appraisal, there are two common errors to avoid. The first is the tendency to want to take over the appraisal and make it a one-way, judgmental appraisal which gives the auxiliary little chance to participate in the discussion. Even if your appraisal is full of compliments and glowing remarks, you have taken away the auxiliary's sense of responsibility for the outcomes and changed the interview from a problem-solving performance appraisal to a superior-subordinate, judgmental interview.

The second error to avoid is the tendency to accept failure to achieve the performance standard as something beyond your control. For example, some dentists are willing to accept a high no-show rate from their patients because they don't feel that they can control the patients' behavior. Among the many possible solutions or combinations of actions that can be taken are: confirming patient appointments, emphasizing to the patients the importance of keeping their appointments so as not to deny treatment to others, and overbooking to reduce the chance of empty time slots. Be sure to take the time to thoroughly examine each problem before giving up.

Summary

The performance appraisal is the next logical step after the planning process and is required to control the performance of the practice and your staff. Preparing for the interview requires participation by both you and the auxiliary to be appraised, plus an administrative system to provide the performance data so that both you and the auxiliary can compare her performance to her performance standards/goals.

The auxiliary should do most of the talking in the interview and brief you on her accomplishment of the performance standards/goals and problem areas encountered. Skillful probing on your part may be necessary to lead the auxiliary to the recognition of some of her performance shortcomings. Remember that criticism seldom improves performance. If the auxiliary cannot be led to recognize her performance problems, you must then assert your authority and insist that she either meet the performance standards or be terminated.

Be thorough and aggressive in tackling the problems and put the results of the interview in writing.

Review Questions

1. List and define the biases that may affect performance appraisal.
2. List the uses for performance appraisal.
3. Using the motivational paradigm $M = f(E \to P) \times (P \to O) V$, explain how the performance appraisal program can increase motivation.
4. Discuss the dentist's personality as it affects performance appraisal.

11
Marketing

Learning Objectives

Upon completion of this chapter, you should be able to:

- Discuss the ethical and legal aspects of advertising as part of a marketing program in the practice of dentistry.
- Explain the use of market segmentation.
- Discuss the difference between internal and external marketing as it applies to dentistry.
- Discuss the use of the *four Ps* in marketing a dental practice.

Introduction

The increase in the supply of dentists relative to the demand for dentistry has created increased competition. With this increased competition, the importance of marketing has grown until it is now probably the most used buzzword in dentistry. The July 1983 Strategic Plan of the American Dental Association recognized the importance of marketing by recommending the following:

- The implementation of "an aggressive and comprehensive ADA marketing program specifically designed to increase utilization."
- "Recognize institutional advertising as an essential element of the above program."
- "Prepare practitioners (existing and future) to be more patient/marketing oriented."
- "Develop continuing education programs to improve dentists' interpersonal skills, marketing strategies and management techniques."

Many dentists dislike marketing because they associate marketing with advertising, which they consider unprofessional. In fact, as we shall see, advertising is only one small part of marketing, and the marketing approach is really a very ethical way of looking at the practice of dentistry.

Some marketing experts define marketing as a system of activities designed to identify the needs and wants of the customer and to design means to meet those needs and wants in a way which will result in a profit. In your case, it means to identify and satisfy the needs and wants of your patients in a way which will allow your practice to meet its responsibilities to the patient, the staff, and yourself.

Put very simply, marketing is the actions you must take to attract and keep patients.

In its broadest sense, marketing covers all the subjects that we discuss in this book. If you look at all your practice functions, from long-range planning to patient management in terms of their impact on patient satisfaction, you are practicing marketing in your practice. The difference lies in the perspective: The patient now becomes the center of attention so that management is viewed from the perspective of its effect on your patients.

The Marketing Plan

When we first discussed planning, we looked at our goals, objectives, and assumptions with little thought about our patients except to forecast some demographic changes such as the aging population and perhaps the population shifts from the north to the Sunbelt. Under the marketing plan concept you must be much more specific about your patients, asking such questions as:

- Who are my patients? (What economic class or classes do they come from?)
- Where do they live?
- What are their needs for dentistry? (How can I change those needs into wants?)
- Do I have the right numbers and kinds of patients? (If I don't have the right numbers and types, where should I look to remedy the situation?)

Market segmentation

Once you have the answers to these questions, you can proceed to the second step in the marketing plan, known as *market segmentation*. Because you have limited resources (as have all businesses), you cannot meet the needs of all the available population. For example, you cannot provide care 24 hours a day; you must decide on the optimum office hours. The optimum time for one segment of the population is seldom the optimum time for other segments. For example, a population of high-income retirees might respond to almost any reasonable hours that you decide upon. Families with small children and both parents working might respond to weekend and evening hours when one parent could care for the children while the other visits your office.

Markets may be segmented on an almost unlimited set of criteria: age, sex, race, social class, education, etc. These criteria in turn are indicators of different needs and wants. Your purpose is to identify a segment of the available population whose needs and wants can be satisfied by what you have to offer.

Toothpaste marketing is one of the best illustrations of target market segmentation. Here marketing experts aimed specific appeals at various target segments based upon the identified wants of each of three target market segments:

1. Children who were attracted to toothpaste primarily by its taste were targeted by Aim® toothpaste, whose ads claimed that children loved the taste of their toothpaste.
2. Pepsodent® and Ultra-Brite® targeted teenagers and young people who had a need to be socially acceptable and attractive, with ads emphasizing the ability of the product to make their teeth whiter and more attractive.

3. Another identified segment consisted of large families who worried about the cost of dental care. Crest® targeted this segment by emphasizing the cavity prevention properties of their toothpaste with the famous slogan "Look ma, no cavities!"

In this case, three segments were identified — children, teenagers, and heads of large families. These segments were not identified primarily because they were children, teenagers, or parents. They were identified because each of these segments have different wants and needs which could reliably be predicted. Children wanted taste, teenagers wanted social acceptance, and the parents wanted to save money.

With few exceptions, patients prefer to choose their dentist from among those who are located close by. Because of this, you are limited in the size and diversity of the market segments available.

For example, social class is a frequent basis for market segmentation, but unless you are in one of the larger cities, it is unlikely that all of the social classes will be available for targeting. The upper-upper class, which comprises only 0.5 percent of the population, are found in a limited number of locales. In some of the rural communities you may be limited to only the lower-middle and the upper-lower social classes.

Experts in consumer behavior maintain that it is not possible to meet the needs and wants of more than two different social classes at the same time — and even then the two social classes must be adjacent, such as the lower-upper class and the upper-lower class.

Once your target market has been identified, you must plan to *promote* your practice with this segment in terms of *product* (service) at suitable *prices* in a *place* which is convenient and attractive. Marketers refer to Promotion, Product, Price, and Place as the *four P's of marketing*, which are combined into a *marketing mix* designed to appeal to the market segment.

Product

It is tempting to say that your product is quality dentistry, for that is the traditional product-oriented approach used for years by many dentists. This approach is characterized by the idea that all a successful dentist must do is produce "quality" dentistry.

This approach is not effective today, because not only does the public resist this approach, but it places undue stress on most dentists when they have to face the ethical decision of whether to offer alternative treatment plans to patients who will not accept what the dentist feels is best for them.

People buy products as an indirect means of attaining higher order satisfaction. As you have seen, patients seldom want quality dentistry; rather, they seek dental care because, among other things, they want to be free from pain, want to be attractive, want prestige, or want to be able to enjoy good food. You are not competing so much with other dentists by producing quality dentistry as you are competing against other things that the patient perceives as a means for attaining those higher order needs.

For the person who wants prestige, you are competing with name brand clothing, jewelry, and Cadillacs. For the person who wishes to be attractive, you are competing with cosmetics, plastic surgeons, and wig makers. Many dentists have realized that the reading materials in the reception room may be self-defeating, for it is very difficult to convince a patient that he needs a $500 treatment plan when he has just been convinced by the ads in your magazines that he really needs that $500 stereo component.

The fact of the matter is that patients are very ill-equipped to evaluate the quality of the dentistry, but they can all evaluate how well they are treated.

Some of the more forward-looking members of the dental profession complain about the narrowness with which most dentists view their product — namely the preoccupation with restorative dentistry — when surveys indicate that the incidence of caries is declining rapidly. These dentists maintain that the product emphasis should be on periodontics and cosmetic dentistry.

Price

Pricing will be discussed in financial terms in Chapter 14. In marketing, you should consider price as the total cost to the patient. The hardest patient costs for some dentists to realize are the psychological ones.

For many patients, the thought of a visit to the dentist causes fear and anxiety, which are further heightened by a seemingly uncaring attitude on the part of the dentist and staff. Another psychological cost to the patient is the loss of self-esteem due to uncaring or inefficient dental staff members, who keep the patient waiting for long periods in the reception room, and the dentist who talks down to them.

Among the real costs are the time lost from work, transportation costs, and the actual cost of treatment. It is unethical to require the patient to pay high prices for quality dentistry when the high costs are due to inefficiencies in the dental practice. The successful dentist must give considerable thought to ways to reduce both the psychological and the real costs of dentistry.

Place

Place as one of the four Ps is, broadly speaking, the availability of services. The factors to consider in the location of the practice have been discussed in Chapter 2, "Locating Your Practice," but we have not discussed place from the viewpoint of the physical availability and appeal of the facility to the target segment.

In past years, the dentist decided on the hours of practice with little regard for the desires of the patients. That has changed with the increased competition for patients. Practice hours must now be based upon the desires of the patients. With the high percentage of working women in the labor force, many dentists are setting their office hours based upon the off-work hours of the patients.

As for the facility itself, before you decorate, take a little time to find out what the decorators know about your target segment and what sort of decor appeals to them. There appear to be certain things that apply to all patients, such as color schemes in blue and green being more peaceful than red, and interesting reading materials reducing the unpleasantness of waiting. Attractive lighting schemes, comfortable seating, and visual contact with the receptionist are basic to a successful practice.

Promotion

Promotion is aimed at letting people know that you are there and that you can meet their needs. In more detail, promotion is designed to move your patients through what is known as the *hierarchy of effects.*

1. From unawareness that you exist to awareness;
2. To an interest in the services you have to offer;
3. To a decision to use your services;
4. To the first visit;
5. To becoming a regular patient whenever the need arises;
6. To becoming your agent by recommending you to friends and acquaintances.

The steps required to move the patient through the hierarchy of effects to the point of the first visit are a function of external promotion. After the patient has entered the office, further movement of the patient through the hierarchy is a function of internal promotion or personal selling on the part of you and your staff.

It is the external promotion which has been most controversial among dentists and other professionals because advertising is one of the elements of external promotion.

Advertising may be defined as publicity received by paying another person for it. The techniques of advertising are complex and beyond the scope of this book except for a brief discussion of the importance of complying with federal, state, and local dental society guidelines governing the content of advertising. The requirements are both legal and ethical ones.

The legal aspects are enforced by consumer legislation and the Federal Trade Commission, which deals with fraud and willful misrepresentation of products or services to the public. The ethical issues are more difficult to determine. After reading the guidelines of several state dental societies, I would recommend that you submit your first attempt at advertising to your local society for comment prior to publication.

However, advertising is not the only part of external promotion. Other means of obtaining publicity are available through public relations and community service. In these cases, the publicity is received without payment on your part. This type of publicity is, of course, harder to control than advertising, since the media must be convinced that your item is newsworthy.

Being active in community service is not only an ethical responsibility, but also a source of exposure to the public through the news media and through personal contact with members of the community. Joining community service organizations, serving as scout counselor, little league sponsor, or in local government quite often result in publicity in the local newspapers and are excellent ways of becoming known to prospective patients and building a positive public image. Still another way of generating favorable publicity is by making yourself available to your local dental society's speaker bureau (if they have one).

While external promotion is important and can provide practice growth, it is probably secondary in importance to internal promotion. If internal marketing is successful in moving patients through steps three to six of the hierarchy of effects, it is possible to sustain practice growth without advertising through new patient referrals to your practice by satisfied regular patients, and by the maintenance of an effective recall system.

Effective internal promotion retains present patients and gains new patients through referrals by maintaining a practice environment that meets the needs and wants of the patients. It combines the elements of product, place, and price and adds the element of patient relations. Besides the elements already discussed, such as reducing the psychological costs of being your patient, we must also add positives such as communicating with the patients in a manner which makes them feel special, as though the practice exists solely for them.

To develop the kind of patient relations that make the patients feel that the practice exists just for them requires efficiency in the delivery of dental care, which we discuss throughout this book, *plus* the application of social psychology to the patient relations. Remember that in the chapter on interviewing we stressed the importance of the first impression bias. The same bias operates on the new patients. The telephone contact with your receptionist is generally the first contact with the practice, and the patient will be trying to confirm the impression formed in that first contact in all subsequent contacts.

It is crucial that you choose a receptionist whose telephone and personal presence project just the right mixture of professional efficiency and human compassion to meet the wants of your target segment. Each member of the staff that the new patient meets must build on the initial positive image presented by the receptionist.

The molding of a staff that can meet the psychological wants of the patients is a difficult one, calling for constant alertness on your part. There are staff members who show one face to you and quite another to the patients in your absence. Frequent random sampling of patient satisfaction by anonymous questionnaires is about the only way to identify a staff member who is rude or unprofessional. Most patients will seek another dentist or react by becoming problem patients before they will tell you about a rude staff member.

Summary

The increasing competition for patients has forced the dentist to become more business oriented in order to survive. This new orientation has caused the dentist to turn to marketing as one of the ways to maintain or increase his patient pool. Because it is so often associated with advertising, marketing has been shunned by dentists in the past. Now, however, dentists are beginning to realize that advertising is only a very small portion of marketing. They see that developing a mix of price, product, place, and promotion into a marketing plan which will provide dentistry which meets the needs and wants of their patients is not only good business but an ethical responsibility as well.

Review Questions

1. Define the term *marketing*.
2. List and define the four Ps of marketing and explain how they can be applied to a dental practice.
3. Explain market segmentation and how it is used in marketing.
4. Explain the difference between advertising and publicity.

12
Patient Management

Learning Objectives

Upon completion of this chapter, you should be able to:

- Discuss how your philosophy affects the patient management program.
- Discuss methods of dealing with problem patients.
- Discuss the factors to be considered when setting up appointment procedures.

The Purpose of Patient Management

The purpose of the patient management system in the dental office is to reduce the unproductive use of time and stress, which will increase the quality and quantity of dental care delivered to the patients. It should be readily apparent that quality dental care cannot be delivered when you and your staff are under conditions of continuous stress. Adequate time must be allotted for each dental procedure to be performed. By creating a controlled flow of patients through the dental practice, the patient management system provides the optimum utilization of resources in terms of time and effort.

An effective patient management system will promote practice growth through satisfied patients by preventing undue delays spent in the reception room, and once in the operatory, will provide for maximum efficiency in executing the dental procedures. The importance of eliminating waiting time in the reception area cannot be overemphasized. In a recent survey, 66 percent of the dental patients mentioned some aspect of time when discussing their dentist.

Requiring the patient to spend excessive time in the reception area is a nonverbal message from you and your staff that is interpreted by the patient as a lack of concern for his/her welfare. It often results in a definite lowering of the patient's self-esteem and his opinion of your practice. This is particularly true if no attempt is made to keep the patient aware of what is going on and the reasons for the delay. You and your staff should consider the appointment as a commitment between you and the patient. It is equally important that the patient be made aware of his/her responsibility to meet the appointment, for if the patient fails to keep the appointment or is late, other patients are denied optimum service.

Philosophy of Patient Management

There is no one ideal management system. The system will vary with the size and nature of the practice and with the philosophy of the dentist. There are, however, certain general principles which will be discussed. Before opening your practice, you should write your philosophy of patient management as a separate part of the office manual. This philosophy will be dynamic and will be revised often as you gain experience and a better understanding of the needs of your practice and the patient. A properly written philosophy will prevent duplication of effort among the staff and the conflicts that arise from such duplication. In the next few paragraphs, we will discuss some of the general decisions you will have to make about patient management.

You must decide how far in advance to schedule patients. To the new dentist, the answer might seem to be very simple — "as far as possible."

However, there are several factors to be considered. First, one of the secrets to practice growth is the ability to accept new patients quickly (some experts estimate that a practice must replace 30 percent of the patient pool each year). Obviously, if patients are scheduled solidly for six weeks in advance, the earliest the average new patient can be seen is around six weeks. Unless there is no other alternative, patients will seldom wait that long for an appointment.

Secondly, there must be some allowance for redos and staff illness. If the schedule is booked solid based upon no errors and a full staff, any deviation can increase staff stress by forcing them to do more in less time and result in longer waiting times for the patient. In general, definite appointments should not be made more than two weeks in advance, and the schedule should not be completely filled for more than two days in advance. This will allow maximum flexibility for your staff and provide the most effective dental care delivery.

The length of the appointment is another major consideration in the patient management system. The objective here is to achieve the maximum efficiency of the staff consistent with the needs of the patient. For example, especially in operative dentistry, quadrant dentistry is the most efficient approach. However, not all patients can accommodate the longer appointments required. The very young and the older patients may require shorter appointments. The following list of representative times is an example of the savings resulting from quadrant dentistry:

greeting and seating the patient	5 minutes
anesthesia and rubber dam	10 minutes
one surface restoration	20 minutes
releasing the patient	10 minutes
total time	45 minutes

Twenty-five minutes of the total time are what might be called overhead time, in that they are required for each patient regardless of the number of restorations accomplished.

In this case, the actual procedure for which fees are charged occupied only 44 percent of the total time, while the preparation and dismissal required the remaining 56 percent of the time. If one more one-surface restoration were accomplished in the same quadrant, this would add an additional 20 minutes to the productive time. Now 62 percent of the visit has been devoted to productive procedures while the overhead time has been reduced to 38 percent.

It is also important to consider *prime times*. These are large blocks of time set aside in the schedule for the more difficult and complex procedures. Other shorter appointments are fitted in around these times. It is important to schedule these prime times when you and the staff are the most productive. Some individuals are most productive in the mornings, while others do not really wake up until the afternoon. The more complex procedures, or prime times, should be scheduled with this consideration in mind, and the simpler procedures such as new patient visits and recalls scheduled outside of peak times.

Once the philosophy of patient management has been developed and presented to your staff, there must now be a way of transmitting information to the staff (particularly to the receptionist) about the procedures and times required for individual patients. This is accomplished by the development of the appointment plan, which is in turn extracted from information contained in the treatment plan.

The Appointment Plan

A typical appointment plan is shown in Figure 12-1. Note that the appointment plan provides a sequence for the treatments, indicates what will be accomplished on each visit, the staff member required and the amount of time required by that staff member. Normally, the units of time are in 15 minute increments; however, some dentists use 5 or 10 minute units. The smaller the unit, the more precise the planning required and the less room for error. The number of units required for each procedure is obtained by maintaining data indicating the average times required for the procedure to be accomplished. (Normally, the longer such data are kept, the more accurate they become and thus permits the use of smaller time units.)

As can be seen from Figure 12-1, the time units column contains the following symbols: 1/2/1. This is a common shorthand for designating the staff and the dentist time required. The first 1 indicates that a dental assistant will be required to greet and seat the patient prior to the arrival of the dentist in the operatory. The 2 indicates that the dentist will be working with a dental assistant for an additional two units, after which the dentist will leave the patient with the dental assistant for an additional one unit of time to accomplish the remainder of the procedure. By referring to this information, the receptionist can schedule the patients. The appointment plan also provides additional information to the receptionist by indicating phone numbers, the best time for phone contact, and the preferred times for appointments.

APPOINTMENTS NECESSARY for DENTISTRY

SCHEDULE FOR Mr. J. J. Jones   TELEPHONE 392-6892
TIME PREFERRED Friday PM   DATE 09-27-82

TIME NECESSARY	SERVICES PLANNED	DAYS BETWEEN APPTS.	DATE & TIME APPOINTED	SERVICES NOT COMPLETED	TIME NECESSARY
1/1/1	26 MO, 27 MOD	5			
1/3/1	12 OL, 13 MO, 14 DO	10			

FORM 78   PROFESSIONAL BUDGET PLAN, MADISON, WISCONSIN   PRINTED IN U.S.A.

Figure 12–1 Appointment plan

The Appointment Book

The first step in preparing the appointment book is to block out those times which are not available for patient treatment, such as lunch, staff meetings, continuing education, and vacations. In addition, some dentists prefer to have short buffer periods built into the day to absorb the unexpected. Among these are the provisions for emergency treatment. Many

134   PATIENT MANAGEMENT

dentists provide for a 30 minute period immediately before lunch for this purpose. If emergencies occur, the lunch hour acts as a buffer for the regular patients. If the emergency is complicated, the dentist compensates with a shorter lunch. A record of the emergency period utilization should be kept to determine if the period is being underutilized, resulting in an unnecessary loss of productivity. If so, you may wish to schedule a longer prelunch appointment and give up your lunch time for the rare emergency patient.

The Recall System

The recall system is another very important element of the patient management system. Very few practices can survive without an effective recall system; nor can you meet your ethical responsibility to provide high-quality dental care to patients without such a system. The recall system provides for planned reentry for treatment of patients who have been out of the active patient category for several months for any number of reasons such as financial problems, or simply because treatment has been completed. The recall system provides a means for checking the status of completed procedures, and for normal preventive recall.

Some dentists schedule the recall at the last appointment, which does save some administrative work and the cost of mailing the recall notice. However, keep in mind the disadvantages of scheduling that far in advance. With advance scheduling for the six-month recall, it is possible that the recall patients will be dominating the patient management system.

Other dentists prefer to mail or call the patient during the month in which the recall visit is due. This can be done by simply noting the recall date in the patient's dental record and placing a recall card in a file indexed by month. This provides for both a by-month and by-patient reference to the recall date.

Some dentists also have the patient address the recall notification card in her own handwriting at the last visit. In these times when there is so much junk mail, patients often throw the majority of the mail in the trash without reading it. However, as they seldom see mail addressed in their own hand, it may increase the possibility that they will read the notice.

The recall system should also provide for recording the number of times the patient was contacted in order to trace the patient who refuses the recall. After two or three attempts to have the patient respond to the recall, a letter should be sent assuring the patient that you will be available in case of need, but that he will be placed in the inactive file unless he responds within a certain period of time. This helps to prevent the possibility of patient abandonment.

The Problem Patient

The problem patients must also be considered in the patient management system. These are patients who consistently fail to keep appointments or are late for them. It is important to impress upon the patient his responsibility for meeting the appointments promptly, or calling in advance when a cancellation becomes necessary. It is often advisable to schedule the chronically late patient a corresponding amount of time prior to the actual appointment.

There is little that can be done for the chronic no-shows other than to suggest that they go on the call list, seek treatment elsewhere, or that they may be scheduled on standby status, and that you will see them only in the event of another cancellation or no-show. It is important to keep track of the cancellation/no-show rate and of the times when they are most likely to occur. Consideration should then be given to adjusting the scheduling philosophy to cope with these problems. For example, when the no-show rate is high, it is unwise to schedule long appointments because of the high probability that the patient will not show up, leaving a long, unproductive period in the day's schedule. Another way of coping with a high no-show rate is to develop a *quick call* list. This is a list of patients who can come for treatment on short notice and can be used to fill in last-minute cancellations and no-shows.

The Role of the Receptionist

The patient management system revolves around the receptionist, and you must give her the authority required to make the system operate. She must have the authority to schedule your work and that of the staff as necessary to provide for effective dental care delivery. While in many cases the receptionist is not senior to the other members of the staff, the receptionist actually is directing and assigning work to the staff. Unless you make it clear to the staff that she has the authority, there is a strong possibility that the other members of the dental staff will resent her efforts to direct their work.

The receptionist must know the skills and capabilities of each member of the staff if scheduling is to be done effectively. It is equally important that certain members of the staff be trained as backup for the receptionist in the event of illness and other absences from the practice. The loss of the receptionist without a knowledgeable backup can cause pandemonium in an otherwise effective practice.

Summary

The patient management system, then, is a critical part of your practice. It consists of a written philosophy and procedures detailing how the appointments should be made, an appointment plan furnishing details of staff requirements, an appointment book in which to schedule the patient treatment and to control patient flow, and a recall system designed to check the reliability of procedures accomplished and to establish a preventive program.

Review Questions

1. Explain how the concept of *prime time* is used in patient management.
2. Describe what items should be included in your philosophy of practice as it applies to patient management.
3. Discuss the administrative considerations involved in setting up a recall system.

13
Office Recordkeeping

Learning Objectives

Upon completion of this chapter, you should be able to:

- Describe the flow of information through the office recordkeeping system.
- Describe the pegboard accounting system.
- Discuss the use of credit and the means of financing dental care.
- Describe the types of dental insurance.
- Describe the use of the usual, customary, and reasonable criteria for setting allowable insurance payments.

The Office Recordkeeping System

Information flow

The office recordkeeping system is really another communications system which passes information back and forth between the dentist and the dental staff, and between the practice and the accountant for control and tax purposes.

Figure 13–1 illustrates the flow of information through the recordkeeping system. Starting at the top of the figure, patient care is rendered, and the information concerning the service rendered then follows two separate but interrelated paths. The left path concerns itself with the dental care and the right path concerns itself primarily with financial data.

At step 2, the left path provides the record of services rendered in the form of progress notes, treatment plans, and other data contained in the dental record. When required, information from this record is transferred to a third-party insurance form as a claim. The services rendered are also summarized on a periodic basis at steps 8 and 11, where they may be analyzed by the dental staff for the purposes of controlling and improving the quantity and quality of dental services within the practice.

The right path furnishes financial data at step 3, which are recorded in individual patient ledgers. The data at this step are used to insure that the practice is compensated by the individual patient for services rendered. From this patient ledger, data are furnished to the third-party claim in the form of fees at step 4.

If the patient does not pay the full amount of the fee at the time of treatment, the patient ledger card forms the basis for billing the patient periodically at step 5 until the account has been paid. As payments are received from third-party claims, in cash or by check as a result of billings, the patient's ledger is updated and passed to the daily summary while the cash and checks are deposited in the practice bank account (step 7) and recorded in the checkbook (step 9). Step 10 usually consists of two ledgers: one for recording revenues or incoming money and a disbursement ledger for recording payments for expenses such as taxes, salaries, rent, and supplies. The data from steps 10, 11, and 12 are then summarized for tax purposes and analyzed as a means of controlling the practice.

The system looks simple, and it is — provided the necessary discipline is maintained to prevent deviations from the office procedure, and office procedures are carefully prepared and disseminated. Consider the number of entries made by the various members of the staff, all of which must be done correctly if the system is to work.

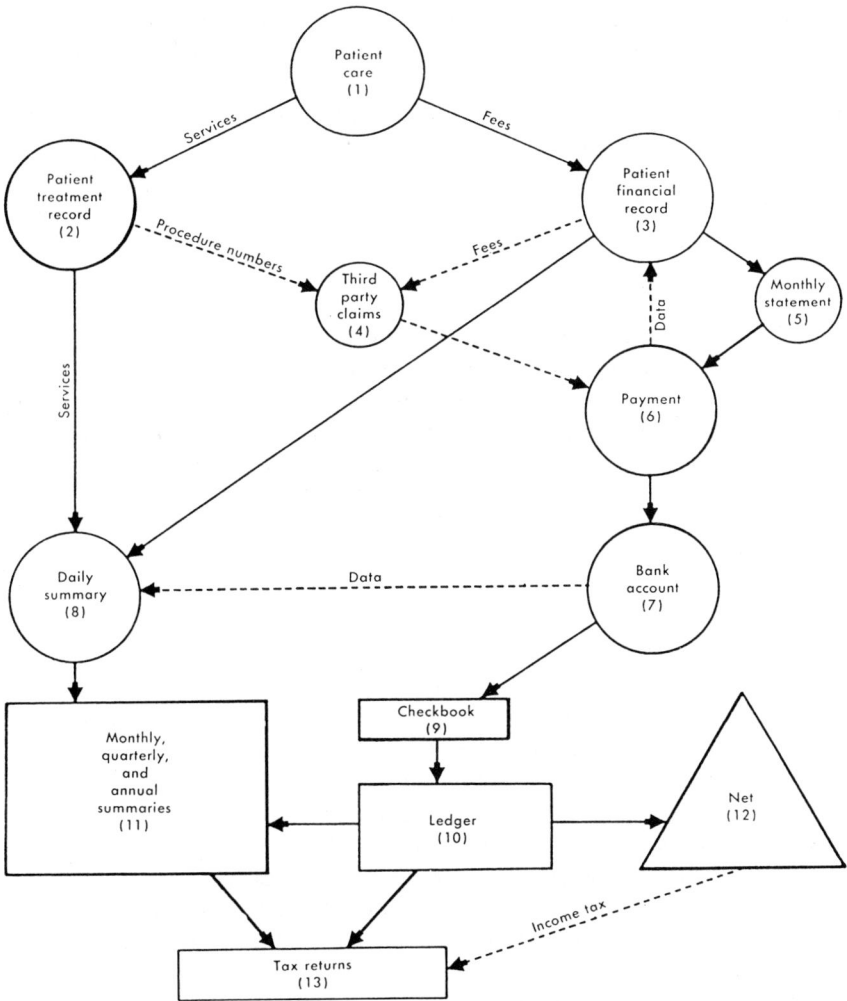

Chart showing interrelationships of components of accounting system for dental offices.

Figure 13–1 Interrelationship of accounting system components for dental offices

You, the dentist, must prepare a treatment plan to be implemented by the receptionist through the appointment book. You and your assistants must accurately prepare the progress notes and record services on a minimum of three forms: the progress notes, the treatment plan, and the note which goes to the receptionist. The receptionist must enter the fees into the daily ledger, account for any payments received, see that the daily ledger and the patient's ledger agree, and provide the patient with a receipt plus make another appointment if necessary. She must then reconcile the cash and checks received with those shown on the ledger and prepare a deposit slip for the bank. All these steps must be followed accurately and systematically. In order to work, the system must be simple and understandable, must provide for a complete record of all that happens, be relatively inexpensive, and contain a system of checks and balances to detect and correct errors.

The pegboard accounting system The *pegboard accounting system* is the most commonly used system in non-computerized dental and medical practices. This system is sometimes referred to as a *one-write* system because a single entry by the receptionist provides the same data to the daily ledger sheet, the patient's ledger card, the patient's receipt or bill as the case may be, and sometimes to the third-party claim form. Obviously, the fewer times the data have to be entered into the system, the fewer chances for error.

The pegboard system is provided by a large number of dental and medical supply companies, and all systems are basically the same with the cost varying widely, mainly depending upon the additional features in the system and whether or not a sales/consulting staff is used. Those with the basic system and no sales/consulting staff are the cheapest. While the systems are all basically the same, they are seldom interchangeable because of the design of the forms and the pegboard itself.

The pegboard system (Figure 13–2) consists of a *pegboard*, which is a board containing a series of pegs used to align the various forms, and a *day sheet*, which records the patient's name, services rendered, fees charged, money received, and remaining balance. The day sheets have varying amounts of other functions available such as deposit slips and additional columns for analyzing the data such as production per doctor. All day sheets have provisions for double-checking accuracy or performing a *proof of posting*.

Aligned over the day sheet are a series of serially numbered receipts and receipt stubs (Figure 13–3). The stub is used to record the patient's name and balance due, after which the stub is normally attached to the dental record for your information prior to the patient's arrival in the operatory. Once treatment is completed, you should indicate the services rendered and the charges, and note if there are any special arrangements for the next appointment.

The patient is then asked to take the stub to the receptionist. If the patient pays, the receptionist then aligns the patient's ledger card with the

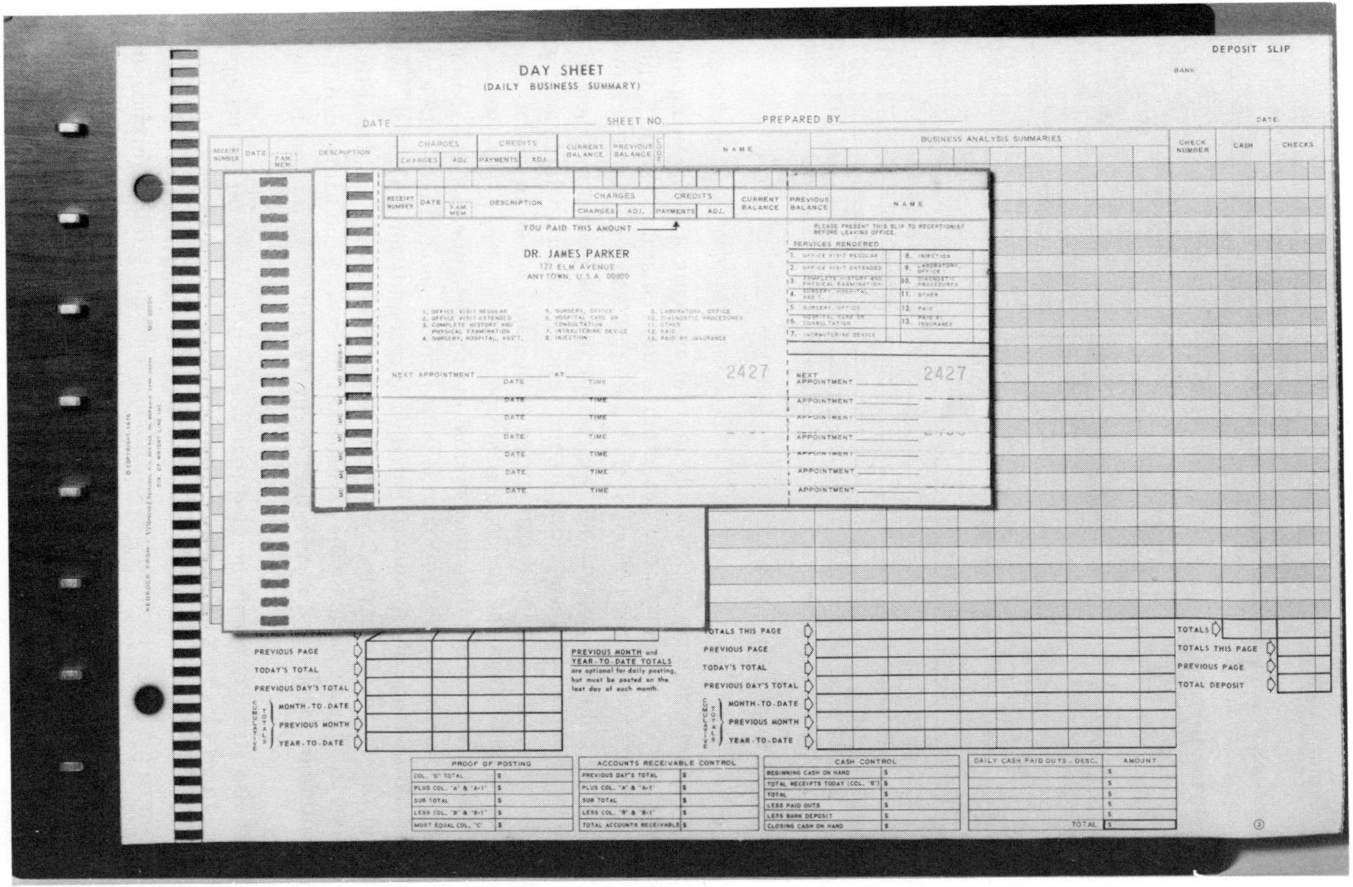

Figure 13-2 Pegboard system

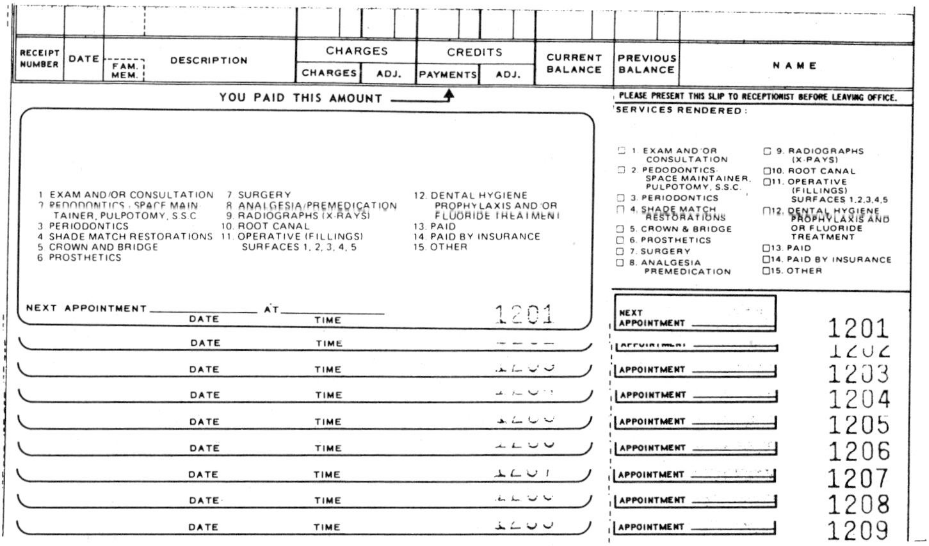

142 OFFICE RECORDKEEPING

Figure 13-3 Receipts

appropriate receipt form on the daily journal and enters the appropriate data as to services rendered, charges, credits, and remaining balance. This receipt is then given to the patient. If the patient asks to be billed, the same procedure is followed except that the receipt now is placed in a self-addressed envelope and given to the patient as the first billing which, among other things, saves the practice the price of postage. When payments are received by mail, the same procedure is repeated.

While embezzlement does happen too often to be ignored in the dental practice, by far the biggest problem is poor bookkeeping due to a lack of firm procedures and discipline. Note that each receipt is serially numbered and that the serial number is transposed to both the ledger card and the day sheet so that all parts of the transaction now bear the same identification number. You must insure that every receipt is accounted for by number.

It is also strongly recommended that you write the fee on the receipt stub or *superbill* which the patient gives to the receptionist. This will prevent the receptionist from being able to collect a higher fee from the patient, entering a lower fee into the journal and pocketing the difference. It is also recommended that the temptation to save money by shortcutting the procedures be avoided. Even in the early days of the practice when only one or two patients are seen in one day, a new day sheet should be used each day. Further, every patient entered in the appointment book should be entered in the daily journal, even if the patient is a cancellation or a no-show. Such procedures will insure that practice income can be easily and accurately accounted for.

Each month those patients with outstanding balances must be billed. There are several ways of accomplishing this billing, all but one of which involves copying the patient ledger card. The ledger cards may be xeroxed by taking them to a store that has a copier, buying a copier for the office, or hiring a company to come to the office to do the copying and mailing of the billings.

Taking the ledger cards out of the office is never a good practice, but in the very early days of the practice it may be the only affordable alternative. Buying a copier is not recommended in the early days of the practice when cash flow is a serious consideration. Using the services of a billing company is a relatively inexpensive alternative; however, you should insert a few test billings to yourself or the office staff on a random basis to test the speed and reliability of the service.

The last alternative is to use your own computer or a computer service. These services not only prepare and mail all billings, they provide all financial data for analysis on a regular basis. The shortcoming to using a service is the nonavailability of data within the practice between cycles. This is somewhat overcome in some services by providing a very small computer terminal from which a limited amount of real-time information is readily available on all patient accounts.

Other elements of the system Among the other recordkeeping forms required is a disbursement pegboard (Figure 13–4) which records all payments made from your practice. The system consists of a pegboard, a disbursement journal similar to the daily journal, a series of checks similar to the receipts, and, in some systems, a stub preprinted for payroll purposes plus an employee earnings record. With the exception of the preprinted payroll stub, the pegboard operates as a checkbook.

Among the records that will be required are records of recurring payments or *accounts payable* owed to various companies such as suppliers, utilities, etc. (See Table 13–1.) Note the account number at the top of the page, which is an arbitrary identification used to simplify the bookkeeping since it is easier to enter the number rather than the name into the various records. The columns from left to right provide for additional control. They indicate the year, the journal page on which the transaction was logged, and the amount.

144   OFFICE RECORDKEEPING

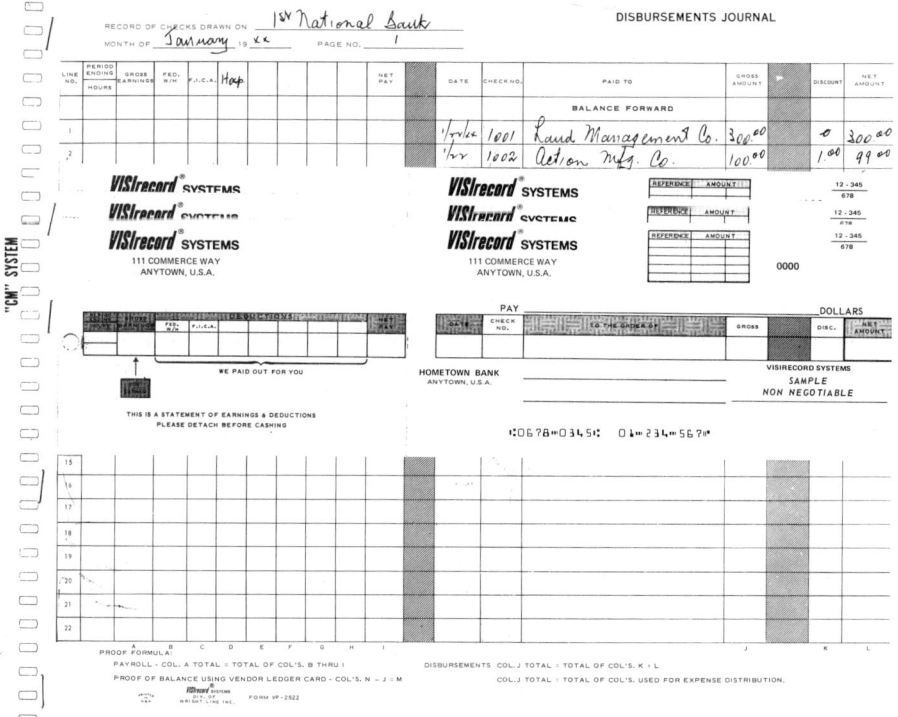

Figure 13-4   Disbursement pegboard

From this document we can see the status of the account with the Michigan Power Company, which indicates that we received an invoice on March 26 for which we have yet to make a payment.

In a similar manner, it is important to keep a record of the depreciation allowed for each item such as dental equipment and the restrictive covenant (see Table 13-2). This record is necessary for tax purposes.

We recommend that you make an occasional random check on the accuracy of the bookkeeping procedures. This can be accomplished by simply making a note of the name and fee charged for each patient. At the end of the day, you may then go over the daily ledger, insuring that there is an entry for each patient and that the entry is correct. All day sheets also have provisions for checking the accuracy of the entries by what is called a *proof of posting*, which simply checks to see that the total charges minus the total payments equal the sum of the patients' current balances. It is very important that you insist that the proof of posting is accomplished without fail and all errors corrected at the end of each day and that funds

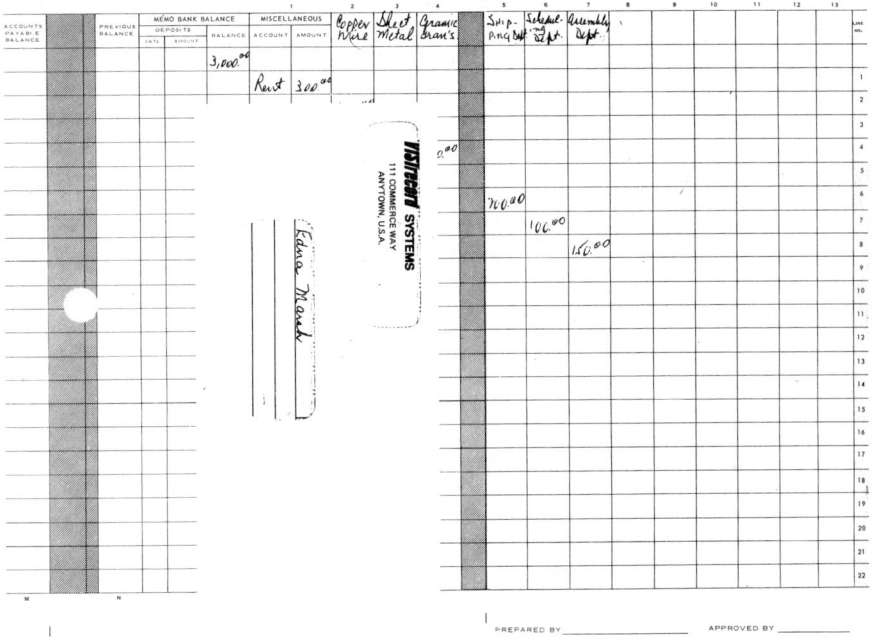

Figure 13-4 (*Cont.*)

are deposited daily in the bank to prevent the risk of theft or embezzlement.

The Use of Credit

There was a time in the past when many dentists bragged that they operated a cash-only practice. However, today our society appears to have accepted the idea that borrowing is no longer socially undesirable, but the American way of life. The dentist who insists on operating a cash practice may not only be denying patients adequate dental care, but may be restricting the growth of the practice.

There are advantages and disadvantages to granting credit in your practice. In most cases, the advantage is that it may encourage patients to avail themselves of treatment they might otherwise forego or delay and increase your patient flow.

Table 13-1 Accounts payable record, electrical power (Michigan Power Co.), acct. no. 301

1965 payments	Journal page	Amount	1965	Invoices rec'd	Journal page	Amount due
			Jan. 17	Dec. serv.	6	$96
Jan. 30 for Dec.	13	$96				0
			Feb. 16	Jan. serv.	21	$105
Feb. 27 for Jan.	30	$105				
			Mar. 16	Feb. serv.	43	$98

Table 13-2 Brown dental unit (depreciation), acct. no. 501

Purchase date	Description	Journal page	Cost	Depreciation	Date
1/1/62	Model no. 345 Brown unit	19	$2,000	$200 (1/10)	12-31-62
				$200 (1/10)	12-31-63
				$200 (1/10)	12-31-64

The disadvantages are:

- Special provisions for controlling A/Rs will increase the time and expense involved in your bookkeeping. (The average cost per patient billing is presently between 65 and 70 cents.)
- Administrative procedures become more complex, requiring that you devise special procedures and policies for handling credit.
- There are additional laws that must be complied with.
- You are denied the alternative uses of the money owed you. It could be used to pay your own debts, thus reducing your interest, or to earn money through investments.

With these drawbacks, it is well to consider whether or not the practice can grow without credit and to use cash discounts to encourage patients to pay when treated. For example, if your investments could earn 15 percent interest, your earnings could be increased by offering a 5 percent discount to non-credit customers. This would give you income to invest at 15 percent, thus earning you 10 percent on funds that might otherwise be tied up in accounts receivable.

Besides the loss of alternative uses for money, there is also the risk of non-collection or bad debts. While the risk will vary between practices and with the varying states of the economy, some researchers have gathered typical collection data indicating how the risk of non-collection varies with time. The typical probability of default is shown below.

> 30 days   3%
> 60 days   6%
> 90 days   10%
> 90+ days 20%
> 6 months 50%

From these data, it is evident that firm, persistent effort must be made to collect accounts receivable as early as possible not only because of the lost alternative uses for the money, but because of the increasing possibility of non-collection as the account ages.

There are several steps that may be taken to reduce the risk of incurring bad debts from your patients:

- When new patients telephone for their first appointment, your receptionist should politely inform them of your policy which requires payment as the treatments are performed.

- When expensive or extensive treatment is required, the receptionist should confer with the patient after the presentation of the treatment plan about the arrangement for payment. Two alternatives are available — the patient may pay as the treatment is rendered, or credit arrangements may be made.
- Limit the patient's payment options after treatment by stating, "Your fee for today is_____. Will you be paying by check or cash?"

If credit arrangements were proposed, the patient's credit should be checked through the use of a credit bureau. As of this writing, the cost of the service is minimal, with fees of $12.00 per month plus $2.50 per credit check. If no information is found, the charge is $1.25.

If the credit report is unfavorable, indicating that the patient is a poor credit risk, the usual approach is for you to inform the patient that you would be delighted to help him, but that services must be on a cash basis. From this point, it is possible in most cases to carry out a treatment plan geared to the patient's ability to pay, even if it does slow down the completion of the treatment.

Credit policies

If credit is unavoidable, A/R problems may be reduced by firm credit policies administered by a motivated office staff. It is important to select a staff member who feels that dentistry is worth every penny charged and who will be both friendly and persistent in her efforts to collect the accounts receivable.

Equally important is the necessity for prompt billing. Normally, routine billings are accomplished for the first two billing cycles (60 days), after which it is a good idea to follow up with telephone calls. The message should never be relayed, but given directly to the patient. The best approach is to ask, "Is there a problem with your bill?" If there is a clinical problem, it is advisable for you to take over and contact the patient immediately for a person-to-person resolution of the problem to maintain good relations with the patient and avoid any possible chance of a malpractice suit.

There are also times when a family may be in a crisis because of illness or other financial problems. An understanding office manager would do well in these cases to set aside collection efforts for 90 days to allow the family to recover from their problems. It is important that when the 90 days are up that collection efforts be resumed immediately with a follow-up telephone call.

Summary of collection actions

Condition	Action
A/R less than 30 days old	Prompt billing.
A/R less than 60 days old	Prompt billing.
A/R more than 60 days	Telephone contact to see if there is a problem.
No results from first telephone call	Telephone to ask patient to come to office so that special arranagements may be made to pay account.
No results from second telephone call	Letter notifying patient of pending legal action

A common answer to the collection phone call is "I was just getting ready to drop it in the mail." If the check is not received within the normal mailing time, another follow-up call should be made immediately. In most cases, if there are no results after two calls, it is common to send a letter stating that if payment is not received within five days, legal action will be taken.

The legal action is to resort either to the small claims court or to a collection agency. There are mixed opinions about the advisability of resorting to either of these options. Many feel that the time and effort involved are not justified by the results.

If you decide to resort to a collection agency, it is important to consider both the company's reputation and their collection methods. Some collection agencies are too aggressive, bordering on illegal harassment in their efforts to force collections. You should also choose a company that will leave certain options open to you, such as returning the patient's account, or settling out of court when requested to do so.

Financing dental care

There are some other considerations in the management of the A/Rs. Some banks will lend money to the patients for dental care without your involvement. Still other banks will loan money to the patient if you will cosign the note. There are both advantages and disadvantages if you cosign the note. You will be paid by the bank as soon as the loan is approved, so there is no delay in receiving payment as there is with the normal A/R procedure. Further, the bank normally assumes the responsibility for making the credit check on the patient, saving you both the time and expense. If the patient should default on the payments, the bank usually will assume the responsibility for collection actions.

The disadvantage, of course, is that if the bank is unable to collect from the patient, you must make good the debt. This arrangement shifts much of the bookkeeping and collection effort from your office to the bank. You may also arrange with many of the major credit card companies to charge dental fees. Your cost will range from 3 to 5 percent of the charges plus the cost of the credit card imprinter, which is minimal.

Dental Insurance Programs

The rapid rise in the number of people covered by dental insurance programs is proving to be both a boon and a curse to dentists. These programs are a boon from the standpoint of increasing the demand for dentistry and a curse because they have increased the complexity of the dentist's management problem. It is possible to have the boon without the curse if you take a little time to understand how the programs work and then apply this knowledge to properly train your office staff.

Types of insurance payments

The broadest category of payments made by someone other than the patient are known as *third-party payments*. Under this title are two major divisions. The first includes those payments made by government agencies at the national, state, or local level in welfare programs, with the major source being the Medicaid program. One source estimated that ten million children are or will be eligible for dental care under this program. While the laws governing the administration of this program vary from the other type of third-party payment we are going to discuss, to you as the dentist the only real difference is in the forms you submit.

The second type of third-party payment, and the one which you will deal with the most, is dental insurance. The latest ADA figures available at this writing indicate that there are four major suppliers under what is known as *Dental Prepayment* or *Dental Insurance* programs. The major supplier is commercial insurance companies, with approximately 27 million beneficiaries. Next in order of size are dental service corporations with about 14 million, Blue Cross and Blue Shield with 4 million, and independent plans with about 3 million beneficiaries.

The dental service corporations known as *Delta Plans* differ in that they are non-profit organizations sponsored by, but separate from, the state dental associations. These organizations are now in all the states plus the District of Columbia. Their purpose is to increase the dental treatment available to the public by lowering the cost of dental care without lowering the quality. Blue Cross/Blue Shield plans are also non-profit organizations which exist in all the states and provide dental insurance either with, or independent of, the Delta Plans.

Though not as large as those previously mentioned, there are two more categories of dental insurance. One is the *closed panel*, which consists of a group of dentists who agree to provide care for groups in return for either a fixed premium or a salary. The important difference between this plan and the other forms of insurance is that this plan does not provide the patient with a choice of dentists. The patient may use only those dentists who are in the panel. The last form is the *self insured trust*, in which the program is managed by the employer or another group which accepts the financial risks of the program.

Provisions of the plans

Now that we know the types of organizations involved, we need to look at the nature of the plans they administer. The coverage provided under these plans varies too widely to do more than provide a general description of the plans. All the plans are what we call *cost-sharing plans* in that the patient and the insurance provider share the cost of treatment. Further, unlimited coverage is very rare, with most plans requiring the patient to bear a portion of the expense in one of five ways.

1. *Deductible.* Under this arrangement, the patient is required to pay a certain portion of the expense of treatment in a given time period before the provider will pay the remainder of the cost. A typical example would be a stipulation that the first 50 dollars per patient or a total of 100 dollars per family per year must be paid by the insured before the provider will start paying the expenses.
2. *Copayment.* In this case, the patient pays a stipulated percentage of the fee and the provider pays the remainder. The percentage of copayment varies between providers and within provider plans by the type of procedure. Normally, the provider shares a larger percentage of the fee for preventive and restorative services.
3. *Maximum Benefit.* This is a feature of most plans. It limits the amount of money the patient can spend on dental treatment. In some cases, the maximum benefit applies to a one-year period and in others, it is a lifetime maximum.
4. *Direct Payment.* This type of plan is usually administered by the employer. After treatment, the patient submits the bill directly to

the employer for reimbursement. There may still be either deductible, copayment, or maximum benefit provisions under this payment method.
5. *Table of Allowance.* Under this system, the provider lists the covered dental procedures and the amount it will pay for each. You must deal with the patient if there is an additional charge.

Having examined the various ways the providers have of sharing and controlling the amount of money they pay to the patient, now look at the methods the providers have for paying the dentist. Just as the providers are concerned about limiting their liability to the patient, they are also concerned about insuring that they have some control over the fees they pay you.

One mechanism is the *usual, customary, and reasonable* fee system. The *usual* fee is the fee that you normally charge your patients for a given procedure. This fee is accepted if it falls within the range of the *customary* fee or the average range of fees charged by other dentists in your area. While the rules change from time to time, at present your fee will be accepted if it falls within the 90th percentile of the customary fee. In other words, your fee will be accepted if it falls within the range of what nine out of ten dentists in your area would charge. If you encounter unusual circumstances, you might charge a higher than normal fee. If the provider felt that this fee was justified under the circumstances, they would pay the higher amount as being *reasonable* under the circumstances.

In the Delta Plan, the basic concept of the usual, customary, and reasonable fee is used, but you are required to pre-file your fee schedule on a confidential basis and agree to accept direct payment. This will not negate your right to receive other payments from the patient such as co-insurance if this is a provision of the plan.

Office procedures

Now that you understand a little about how the system works, how can you set up your office procedures to take advantage of the benefits offered by third-party payments? The first things you will need are the forms for submitting your claims. The ADA has provided a standard form (see Figure 13–5) for this purpose. With the exception of Medicare, the vast majority of the providers will use this form, which greatly simplifies your administrative problems.

We won't go into the mechanics of filling out the form, since the ADA provides an excellent set of instructions with their insurance brochure. The

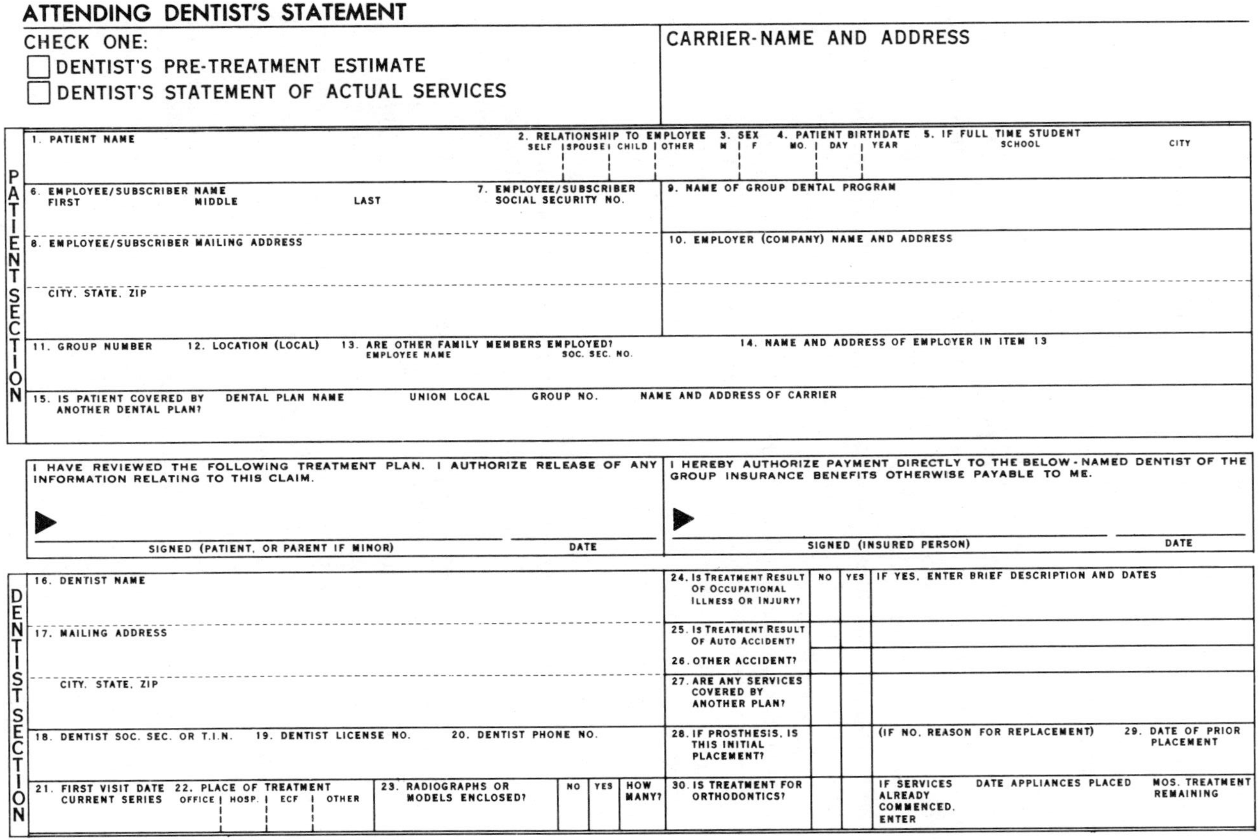

ATTENDING DENTIST'S STATEMENT

CHECK ONE:
☐ DENTIST'S PRE-TREATMENT ESTIMATE
☐ DENTIST'S STATEMENT OF ACTUAL SERVICES

CARRIER-NAME AND ADDRESS

PATIENT SECTION

1. PATIENT NAME
2. RELATIONSHIP TO EMPLOYEE — SELF | SPOUSE | CHILD | OTHER
3. SEX — M | F
4. PATIENT BIRTHDATE — MO. | DAY | YEAR
5. IF FULL TIME STUDENT — SCHOOL — CITY
6. EMPLOYEE/SUBSCRIBER NAME — FIRST — MIDDLE — LAST
7. EMPLOYEE/SUBSCRIBER SOCIAL SECURITY NO.
9. NAME OF GROUP DENTAL PROGRAM
8. EMPLOYEE/SUBSCRIBER MAILING ADDRESS
CITY, STATE, ZIP
10. EMPLOYER (COMPANY) NAME AND ADDRESS
11. GROUP NUMBER
12. LOCATION (LOCAL)
13. ARE OTHER FAMILY MEMBERS EMPLOYED? — EMPLOYEE NAME — SOC. SEC. NO.
14. NAME AND ADDRESS OF EMPLOYER IN ITEM 13
15. IS PATIENT COVERED BY ANOTHER DENTAL PLAN? — DENTAL PLAN NAME — UNION LOCAL — GROUP NO. — NAME AND ADDRESS OF CARRIER

I HAVE REVIEWED THE FOLLOWING TREATMENT PLAN. I AUTHORIZE RELEASE OF ANY INFORMATION RELATING TO THIS CLAIM.
▶ SIGNED (PATIENT, OR PARENT IF MINOR) — DATE

I HEREBY AUTHORIZE PAYMENT DIRECTLY TO THE BELOW-NAMED DENTIST OF THE GROUP INSURANCE BENEFITS OTHERWISE PAYABLE TO ME.
▶ SIGNED (INSURED PERSON) — DATE

DENTIST SECTION

16. DENTIST NAME
17. MAILING ADDRESS
CITY, STATE, ZIP
18. DENTIST SOC. SEC. OR T.I.N.
19. DENTIST LICENSE NO.
20. DENTIST PHONE NO.
21. FIRST VISIT DATE CURRENT SERIES
22. PLACE OF TREATMENT — OFFICE | HOSP. | ECF | OTHER
23. RADIOGRAPHS OR MODELS ENCLOSED? — NO | YES | HOW MANY?

	NO	YES	IF YES, ENTER BRIEF DESCRIPTION AND DATES
24. IS TREATMENT RESULT OF OCCUPATIONAL ILLNESS OR INJURY?			
25. IS TREATMENT RESULT OF AUTO ACCIDENT?			
26. OTHER ACCIDENT?			
27. ARE ANY SERVICES COVERED BY ANOTHER PLAN?			
28. IF PROSTHESIS, IS THIS INITIAL PLACEMENT?			(IF NO, REASON FOR REPLACEMENT) — 29. DATE OF PRIOR PLACEMENT
30. IS TREATMENT FOR ORTHODONTICS?			IF SERVICES ALREADY COMMENCED, ENTER — DATE APPLIANCES PLACED — MOS. TREATMENT REMAINING

Figure 13–5 Attending dentist's statement

important part for you to remember is to see that your receptionist asks the patient if he is covered by insurance, and if so, to have him bring his forms with them. It will also save time if the patient is requested to fill out the top of the form before the appointment.

In filling out the bottom portion of the form, be specific, using the ADA Dental Procedures Codes and the standard tooth numbering system. In addition, it is a good idea on restorative procedures to note the number of surfaces (MOD, etc.) just in case your receptionist inadvertently enters the wrong procedure code. Normally the processor at the insurance company will correct the entry if the additional information is available. It will speed up processing if the receptionist will keep a list of commonly used procedure codes available for quick reference.

Before you present your treatment plan, you or your receptionist must become familiar with the provisions of the patient's policy. To streamline this requirement, you should gather information on all the dental plans that you anticipate being involved with. To gather this information, it usually is better to contact the employer or the group that is covered by the policy rather than the insurance company. The insurance company may have a number of different plans, and the employer will be more familiar with the exact provisions of his particular plan. To record this information in an organized manner, you should use a form similar to the one shown in Figure 13-6 and file the data alphabetically by company.

Note that Figure 13-6 provides information on the scope of the benefits plus the name and phone number of the contact person at the insurance company. Whenever you must deal with the provider, use the phone as much as possible to expedite your claims, and record the name of the person you spoke to for ease of follow-up should it become necessary.

It is imperative that the patient be thoroughly informed about how much of the cost of the treatment plan will be covered by insurance. Never assume that the patient understands the coverage on the policy, since experience indicates that most patients do not. The form in Figure 13-7 should be completed after the patient has been briefed on the treatment plan to serve as a matter of record for both of you.

If the fee for the treatment plan is greater than $200.00 or an amount stipulated by the provider, you must submit a *predetermination* request, which is the same standard ADA form but is checked in a different block at the top of the form. Upon receipt of the form, the provider will determine the patient's eligibility, calculate the benefits payable, and return a copy of the form to you and to your patient. Upon receipt of the form, you may schedule the patient to begin treatment, but again, be certain that you review the benefits if they have changed since the plan presentation.

Company:	Florida Manufacturing Co.
Local Address:	1010 E. 15th St., Melbourne, FL (ph.) 555-1669: Mrs. Joan Fields, Pers. Mgr.
Insurance Co.:	Indemnity Ins. Co.
Send Claims To:	2500 E. Colonial Dr.: Orlando, FL (ph.) 655-1229. (Jane Figit, Claims Supervisor)
Benefits:	Deductible — $25 per year, excluding prophy & x-rays Maximum — $750/year — $5,000 lifetime Co-payment — 80/20: 50/50 on pros. & gold. Miscellaneous — Predetermination necessary over $150. No ortho. or cosmetic dentistry benefits "Optimal Treatment" Provision.

Figure 13-6 Benefits summary form

Now that you understand how to prepare both your patient and your forms for third-party payment, you must set up office procedures to follow up on and expedite the flow of paper to the insurance companies and the flow of money from the insurance companies. A cardinal rule is never to mix your financial records and dental records together. Set up separate files to monitor your insurance process. You should have four separate files: claims awaiting preauthorization, claims awaiting completion of treatment, claims awaiting payment, and payment complete. In addition, you may wish to keep an *insurance summary record,* as shown in Figure 13-8.

With experience, you will know the average time for return of the preauthorization and the payments. Then you may follow up on the delinquent forms by using the insurance summary record to identify the outstanding claims, or set up a suspense file of 3 × 5 cards with the pertinent information. The cards can then be filed in a suspense file labeled by day of the month at appropriate times for follow-up. Remember that the way your office handles this file will have a definite impact on cash flow. If you have a lengthy treatment plan, it may be possible to break the plan into stages and to submit claims for payment as each stage is completed rather than waiting until all treatment is completed.

Your office must have the attitude that cooperation with both the insurance company and the patient is essential to the success of the practice and the welfare of the patient. The patient must be impressed with the fact that he is responsible for the payment of the fees regardless of any arrangements he may have with insurance companies. If you decide to accept direct payment, your office should mail in the completed claim form rather

PATIENT FINANCIAL UNDERSTANDING FORM
(NOT FOR INSTALLMENT PLAN)

DENTIST NAME
AND ADDRESS:

PATIENT NAME
AND ADDRESS:

PARENT:

SERVICES PERFORMED OR TO BE PERFORMED:

DATE OF SERVICES:

1. FEE FOR SERVICES .... $ _____
2. AMOUNT PAYABLE BY INSURANCE OR SERVICE PLAN .... $ _____
3. BALANCE DUE .... $ _____

THE PATIENT (GUARDIAN) AGREES TO BE AND HEREBY IS FULLY RESPONSIBLE FOR TOTAL PAYMENT TO: (DENTIST NAMED ABOVE) OF PROCEDURES PERFORMED IN THIS OFFICE INCLUDING ANY AMOUNTS WHICH ARE NOT COVERED BY ANY DENTAL INSURANCE OR PREPAYMENT PROGRAM THAT THE PATIENT MAY HAVE. BALANCE DUE IS PAYABLE ON:

_____   _____
SIGNATURE OF PATIENT (PARENT IF PATIENT IS A MINOR)   DATE

[ada] 76-1

PATIENT FINANCIAL UNDERSTANDING FORM
(FOR INSTALLMENT PLAN)

DENTIST NAME
AND ADDRESS:

PATIENT NAME
AND ADDRESS:

PARENT:

SERVICES PERFORMED OR TO BE PERFORMED:

DATE OF SERVICES:

NOTE: ALL SPACES SHOULD BE COMPLETED OR MARKED "**NA**" (NOT APPLICABLE).

1. FEE FOR SERVICES .... $ _____
2. TOTAL DOWN PAYMENT .... $ _____
3. CHARGES COVERED BY INSURANCE OR SERVICE PLAN .... $ _____
4. UNPAID BALANCE .... $ _____
5. AMOUNT FINANCED .... $ _____
6. **FINANCE CHARGE** .... $ _____
7. **FINANCE CHARGE EXPRESSED AS ANNUAL PERCENTAGE RATE** .... _____ %
8. TOTAL PAYMENT DUE (5 PLUS 6 ABOVE) .... $ _____
9. TOTAL CHARGES (1 PLUS 6 ABOVE) .... $ _____

"TOTAL PAYMENT DUE" (8 ABOVE) IS PAYABLE TO: (DENTIST NAMED ABOVE) IN: MONTHLY INSTALLMENTS OF $ _____ . THE FIRST INSTALLMENT IS PAYABLE ON: _____ , 19 ____ , AND EACH SUBSEQUENT PAYMENT IS DUE ON THE SAME DAY OF EACH CONSECUTIVE MONTH UNTIL PAID IN FULL.

THE PATIENT (GUARDIAN) AGREES TO BE AND HEREBY IS FULLY RESPONSIBLE FOR TOTAL PAYMENT OF PROCEDURES PERFORMED IN THIS OFFICE INCLUDING ANY AMOUNTS WHICH ARE NOT COVERED BY ANY DENTAL INSURANCE OR PREPAYMENT PROGRAM THAT THE PATIENT MAY HAVE.

_____   _____
SIGNATURE OF PATIENT (PARENT IF PATIENT IS A MINOR)   DATE

[ada] 76-2 (INST PLN)

SEE REVERSE SIDE FOR ORDER INFORMATION

Figure 13–7

PATIENTS NAME	CARRIER	AUTHORIZATION REQUIRED		REQUEST FOR AUTHORIZATION MAILED		AUTHORIZATION RECEIVED			CLAIM FORM MAILED		AMOUNT RECEIVED FROM INSURANCE		AMOUNT PATIENT TO PAY	ARRANGEMENTS FOR PAYING BALANCE
		YES	NO	DATE	AMOUNT	DATE	AMOUNT	CLAIM NO.	DATE	AMOUNT	DATE	AMOUNT		

Form No 274 Professional Budget Plan, Madison, Wisconsin, Printed in U.S.A.

Figure 13–8 Insurance summary record

than leave it to the patient, since the patient is not as interested in your being paid as you are and may delay mailing the forms.

In the event that you do have problems with the insurer, remember to document your transactions and when you do not receive satisfaction, include the insured company, state insurance commissioner, and the ADA as information addressees on your correspondence with the company. This seems to speed up the insurer's reactions considerably. Finally, if all else fails, avail yourself of the peer review mechanism provided by your state dental society. Many of these problems can be eliminated by a well-organized, cooperative approach to the third-party payment program.

Summary

The office recordkeeping system is a key element in determining the success of your practice. Without accurate data on treatment rendered, fees charged and received, and a record of disbursements, you will not only be unable to make informed decisions about your practice and collect the money owed, you will also be vulnerable to malpractice suits and in trouble with the Internal Revenue Service.

There are two major parts to the recordkeeping system: the progress notes and other documentation of treatment rendered, and a separate but coordinated record of fees charged, received and money owed to you. The most commonly used method of recordkeeping is the pegboard or one-write system, which minimizes the number of separate entries required, thus reducing the chance of error.

The system will only operate effectively if you standardize the procedures and maintain strict administrative discipline.

Credit may become as much a way of life in the dental practice as it has in all other phases of American life. You must seriously consider your credit policies in the light of increased competition and be aware of the advantages and disadvantages of granting credit. The major advantage is that granting credit may increase practice growth. The disadvantages are the increased bookkeeping costs, the loss of alternative use of the money while you are waiting to be paid, and the increased risk of bad debts.

Coping with the additional complexities involved in dealing with third-party insurance can be a stressful experience for you, your staff, and your patients. However, if you spend a little time getting familiar with the concepts and procedures involved in these programs and set up an effective administrative system to deal with insurance payments, third-party insurance can help more patients receive the care they need and add to your practice growth.

Review Questions

1. List the parts of the pegboard system and describe how the parts are used in the recordkeeping system.
2. List the different types of records required in your office recordkeeping system, such as progress notes and depreciation schedules.
3. Draw a diagram depicting the flow of information through the dental office recordkeeping system.
4. Discuss the steps in contacting patients who are delinquent in paying their account.
5. Describe the use of the credit bureau.
6. Discuss the criteria for choosing a collection agency.
7. Explain the difference between open and closed panel insurance programs.
8. Explain the difference between deductible payment and co-payment.
9. Define usual, customary, and reasonable fees.

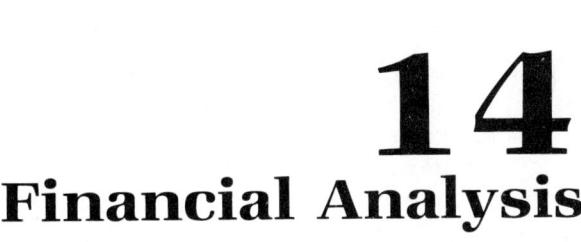

14
Financial Analysis

Learning Objectives

Upon completion of this chapter, you should be able to:

- Describe the elements in the balance sheet and how they reflect the financial status of the dental practice.
- Use financial ratios to conduct vertical and horizontal analyses of the financial status of a dental practice.
- Construct a cash flow budget.
- Describe the principles of and conduct a breakeven analysis.

Introduction

In the last chapter, we looked into the office recordkeeping system, a system designed to gather information on the various facets of a dental practice. We will now see how this information can serve as a basis for making managerial decisions and controlling the practice. By control, we mean the ability to discern deviations from your objectives. You then need to take corrective action either by changing your objectives or changing your plans.

Before we go on, we should look at some of the major causes of business failure and then think about how financial analysis can prevent these things from happening to us. The major causes of business failure are

- not enough patients
- high operating costs
- poor credit or collection policies
- too many fixed assets (operatories, equipment, etc.)

Many managers tend not to get involved in running their business until a major problem develops. Then it's too late for careful analysis and decision making. Remember that managing a practice is not the same as operating a practice. When you are operating a practice, you are treating patients as a member of the dental team. When you are managing a practice, you are making decisions about how to best attain practice objectives. It goes without saying that the more precise and quantifiable your objectives are, the easier it will be to discern deviations. For example, if you say, "My objective is to earn $200 next week," and you earn $198, obviously you have not attained your objective because you're $2 short. There's no question or problem in discerning a deviation in this case.

Financial analysis requires information on each of the practice's important activities, which in turn requires routines and disciplines in recordkeeping. It requires one other thing: a determination of the cost-benefit of the financial data and analyses that you are going to accomplish. You must question the value of the data and analyses. In other words, how much are the data going to cost, and what am I going to do after I get them?

If your financial analyses do not provide you with the data you need to make worthwhile decisions, then you don't need the information. Typical questions answered by financial analysis are: *How profitable are my fees? Are my costs out of line?* and *Do I owe too much money?*

The purpose of this chapter is to enable you to communicate with accountants by understanding basic accounting concepts and to be able to evaluate the cost-benefit ratio of financial information. The cost of financial analysis at the time of this writing varied from $50 to $275 a month. The services provided varied from providing just enough information for income tax preparation to far more data than could actually be used.

The Balance Sheet

Now for a look at some of the tools of financial analysis. Figure 14–1 depicts a balance sheet, which is a financial picture of your practice at a point in time. The balance sheet is divided into two columns with an *as of* date at the top. It is important that you realize that this sheet is only accurate for the instant of the time indicated by the *as of* date. The financial data in the balance sheet are constantly changing over time, as will be seen later.

On the left side of the balance sheet are shown the assets of the practice and on the right side, the liabilities. The difference between the *total assets* and *total liabilities* is known as *net worth*.

Assets are made up of two main categories: *current assets* and *fixed assets*. Current assets are assets which can be readily converted to cash during the accounting period (which is normally the fiscal year). Current assets are listed in order of liquidity, which means in the order of the ease with which they can be converted to cash. Cash in the bank ($15,000) is listed first. The next most easily converted are accounts receivable ($35,000). Next, we have what is called *an accrual,* which is prepaid insurance; until that insurance is actually used up, it is accounted for by storing it in current assets.

The next category of assets are the *fixed assets,* or physical assets

Current assets		Current liability	
Cash	$15,000	Notes payable	$8,000
Accounts receivable	35,000	Taxes	2,000
Prepaid insurance	1,000	FICA	1,000
TOTAL	*$51,000	TOTAL	$11,000
Fixed assets		Long-term liability	
Dental equipment	$75,000	Mortgage	$31,000
Depreciation	(19,000)	School	10,000
	*$56,000	TOTAL	*$41,000
Furniture	6,000	Net worth	*$59,000
Depreciation	($2,000)	TOTAL LIABILITIES	52,000
	* 4,000	Total liabilities	
TOTAL ASSETS	$111,000	+ net worth	$111,000

Figure 14–1 Balance sheet Jan. 31, 1979

required to conduct your practice, i.e., dental equipment with an original cost of $75,000. (All fixed assets are listed at their original cost to you.) Immediately below is the depreciation, which is a way of accounting for fair wear and tear on the equipment. So far, the dental equipment has depreciated $19,000 so that it is really worth only about $56,000. The same depreciation procedures apply to the office furniture which was worth $6,000 when it was new and now has depreciated by $2,000, making it now worth $4,000. The total assets or sum of the current and fixed assets is $111,000.

On the other side of the balance sheet are the *current liabilities*, or those debts which will be due during this accounting period. These are notes payable to creditors (the banks, suppliers, and so forth) of $8,000. There are also current liabilities in the form of $2,000 of income tax and $1,000 of social security withholding for a total current liability of $11,000.

Under *long-term liabilities* (liabilities which will not become due or be paid during this period) are a mortgage of $31,000 and a school debt of $10,000, for a total of $41,000. The *total liabilities* (current plus long-term) sum up to $52,000.

We now come to an important formula: *total assets = liabilities + net worth*. Applying this formula to the data in the balance sheet, we find $111,000 = $52,000 + net worth. Transposing, we find total assets ($111,000) − total liabilities ($52,000) = net worth ($59,000). A closer examination of the balance sheet will reveal the reason for its name. Both sides of the sheet must always be in balance.

Another thing that should be brought out is that we are doing our accounting on an accrual basis rather than a cash basis. Accrual accounting means that the transactions are noted when the commitment is made and not when the cash changes hands. For example, if you order some equipment for $10,000, that amount is subtracted from current assets at the time rather than waiting until the equipment is actually paid for. Similarly, earnings are placed in accounts receivable in the current assets although the money has not yet changed hands. Accounting may also be done on what is called a cash basis. In this case, the balance sheet is changed when cash actually changes hands; however, this system is seldom used and will not be discussed here.

To see how the balance sheet is actually maintained, let us start with the balance sheet as it might exist on the first day of a new practice when we are starting out with nothing. You have no current assets, no total assets, no current liabilities, or net worth.

Let us assume that we borrow $30,000 repayable at $200 per month with payments commencing six months from now. The balance sheet would record the transaction as follows (Figure 14–2). We would enter $30,000 in current assets because we haven't spent it for anything yet. We have no

Assume a loan of $30,000, repayable at $200/month payments commencing six months from now.

Current assets		Current liabilities	
Cash	30,000	Notes payable	1,200
Fixed assets	-0-		
TOTAL ASSETS	30,000	Long-term liabilities	
		Loan	28,800
		Net worth	-0-
		TOTAL LIABILITIES	30,000
		Total liabilities + net worth	30,000

Figure 14-2 Balance sheet

fixed assets because we haven't bought any equipment, so our total assets (current plus fixed) equal $30,000. In the current liabilities (thinking of the full year) we have six monthly payments on the loan for a total of $1,200. We also have a long-term liability of $30,000 minus the $1,200, or $28,800 (because eventually we're going to have to pay back the full loan of $30,000). Using the formula: total assets = total liabilities + net worth, we see that total assets of $30,000 = total liabilities of $30,000; therefore, using the formula, total assets − total liabilities, net worth is 0.

Now assume that 30 days later we have purchased $6,000 worth of office furniture and $12,000 worth of dental equipment (Figure 14-3). Because we have spent $18,000, the current assets and cash have dropped to $12,000. The fixed assets have increased to $18,000, and our total assets remain unchanged. Looking at the liabilities, there haven't been any changes. The long-term liability is still $28,800 plus $1,200 of current liability for a total liability of $30,000. Applying the balance sheet formula, we see that total assets and total liabilities are both $30,000; therefore, net worth still remains 0. There's just no way around it; until some income is earned, net worth will remain 0.

Now assume that you're getting a little hungry, so you decide to draw $2,000 in cash for living expenses (Figure 14-4). This reduces the current assets by $2,000, and while there is no change in fixed assets, the total assets have now dropped to $28,000 but the total liabilities are still $30,000. Applying the balance sheet formula, total assets ($28,000) − total liabilities ($30,000), the net worth is now negative, or −$2,000.

Now assume that we've earned $1,000 for the month, of which $600 is in cash and $400 is in accounts receivable, and that we are going to enter

Purchase $6,000 office furniture and $12,000 dental equipment.

Current assets		Current liabilities	
Cash	12,000	Notes payable	1,200
Fixed assets		**Long-term liability**	
Office furnishings	6,000	Loan	28,800
Dental equipment	12,000		
	18,000	Net worth	-0-
TOTAL ASSETS	30,000	TOTAL LIABILITIES	30,000
		Total liabilities + net worth	30,000

Figure 14–3 Balance sheet

10 percent depreciation on the fixed assets. How does the balance sheet reflect these transactions (Figure 14–5)?

The cash in current assets would increase by $600 and a new heading, accounts receivable, would be added for $400, increasing the total current assets to $11,000. By depreciating the office furnishings by $600 and the dental equipment by $1,200, the fixed assets have been reduced by $1,800 for total fixed assets of $16,200. Adding the two assets together provides new total assets of $27,200.

Current liabilities plus long-term liabilities in the right-hand column still remain at $30,000. Applying the basic formula of assets − liabilities = net worth, there are $27,200 in assets − $30,000 in liabilities = a net worth of −$2,800, reflecting the difference between earnings and depreciation.

Draw $2,000 cash for living expenses.

Current assets		Current liabilities	
Cash	10,000	Notes payable	1,200
Fixed assets		**Long-term liabilities**	
Office furnishings	6,000	Loan	28,800
Dental equipment	12,000		
	18,000	Net worth	(−2,000)
TOTAL ASSETS	28,000	TOTAL LIABILITIES	30,000
		Total liabilities + net worth	28,000

Figure 14–4 Balance sheet

Earn $1,000 for month ($600 cash, $400 A/R)
Add 10% depreciation.

Current assets		Current liabilities	
Cash	10,600	Notes payable	1,200
A/R	400	TOTAL	1,200
TOTAL	11,000	Long-term liabilities	
Fixed assets			
		Loan	28,800
Office furnishings	6,000	Net worth	(2,800)
Depreciation	(600)	TOTAL LIABILITIES	30,000
Dental equipment	12,000	Total liabilities	
Depreciation	(1,200)	+ net worth	27,200
TOTAL	16,200		
TOTAL ASSETS	27,200		

27,200 − 30,000 = (2,800)
(ASSETS − LIABILITIES = NET WORTH)

Figure 14–5 Balance sheet

There was a total increase in current assets of $1,000 and a decrease in fixed assets of $1,800 for an $800 decrease.

Seven months later (Figure 14–6), assume that you have now earned $50,000 of which $20,000 has been received in cash and $30,000 in accounts receivable. This increases cash by $20,000, bringing it up to $30,600, and accounts receivable increases by $30,000, for a total current assets of $61,000. As the fixed assets have already been depreciated for the year, there is no change, so total assets equal $77,200. The current and long-term liabilities remain unchanged for a total of $30,000. Applying the formula: assets − liabilities = net worth, you have $77,200 − $30,000 = $47,200 for net worth.

Now take a look at what happens when you pay off $200 of the notes payable (Figure 14–7). To keep the balance sheet balanced, we must take $200 off the left-hand side and $200 off the right-hand side. It's easy to see that paying the $200 would reduce the notes payable from $1,200 to $1,000. To balance the sheet, it is then necessary to reduce current assets by $200 for the cash spent to pay the loan, making it $30,400. So the total assets have been reduced by $200 to $77,000, and the total liabilities have been reduced by $200 to $29,800. Going back to our formula again, total assets of $77,000 − liabilities of $29,800 equals a net worth of $47,200. Notice that this transaction didn't affect the net worth at all.

You now decide to catch up with your salary by drawing $12,000 over

168 FINANCIAL ANALYSIS

Step 1 Earn $50,000 ($20,000 cash, 30,000 A/R)
Step 2 $200 paid on notes payable
Step 3 Draw $12,000 over the 6 months (drew $2,000 on 1st month)

Current assets		Current liabilities	
Cash	30,600		1,200
A/R	30,400		
TOTAL	61,000		
Fixed assets		Long-term liabilities	
Office furnishings	6,000	Loan	28,800
Depreciation	(600)		
Dental equipment	12,000	Net worth	47,200
Depreciation	(1,200)	TOTAL LIABILITIES	30,000
TOTAL	16,200	Total liabilities	
TOTAL ASSETS	77,200	+ net worth	77,200

$$77{,}200 - 30{,}000 = 47{,}200$$
(ASSETS − LIABILITIES = NET WORTH)

Figure 14–6 Balance sheet

Step 2 — $200 paid on notes payable.

Current assets		Current liabilities	
Cash	30,400	Notes payable	1,000
A/R	30,400	TOTAL	1,000
TOTAL	60,800	Long-term liabilities	
Fixed assets		Loan	28,800
Office furnishings	6,000		
Depreciation	(600)	Net worth	47,200
Dental equipment	12,000	TOTAL LIABILITIES	29,800
Depreciation	(1,200)	Total liabilities	
TOTAL	16,200	+ net worth	77,000
TOTAL ASSETS	77,000		

TOTAL ASSETS − LIABILITIES = NET WORTH
$$77{,}000 - 29{,}800 = 47{,}200$$

Figure 14–7 Balance sheet

the six months (Figure 14–8). This will reduce the cash by $12,000 for a new total of $18,400, while the accounts receivable remain unchanged. The current assets have dropped to $48,000, making the total assets $65,000. Neither current liabilities nor long-term liabilities have changed. Again, applying the formula: assets ($65,000) − liabilities ($29,800) = net worth ($35,200).

This is how the balance sheet operates. It tells you where your assets and liabilities are, and as we'll see when we get into ratio analysis, the balance sheet provides you with some idea of the financial health of the practice.

The Income Statement

The next important tool for financial analysis which will be used more frequently, and which probably is easier to understand, is the income statement. The income statement is also called the operating statement or profit-and-loss statement. Figure 14–9 depicts a simple income statement for the period from January 1 to December 31, so it's actually a summation of what has happened over the past year. It reveals an income of $35,000 and records expenses such as auxiliaries' salaries, $9,000, stationery and postage, $300, dental supplies, depreciation, amortization, office rent, etc.; for a to-

---

Step 3 — Draw $12,000 for last 6 months living expenses.

Current assets		Current liabilities	
Cash	18,400	Notes payable	1,000
A/R	30,400	TOTAL	1,000
TOTAL	48,800		
Fixed assets		Long-term liabilities	
Office furnishings	6,000	Loan	28,800
Depreciation	(600)	Net worth	35,200
Dental equipment	12,000	TOTAL LIABILITIES	29,800
Depreciation	(1,200)	Total liabilities	
TOTAL	16,200	+ net worth	65,000
TOTAL ASSETS	65,000		

TOTAL ASSETS − LIABILITIES = NET WORTH
65,000 − 29,800 = 35,200

Figure 14–8 Balance sheet

John Smith, D.D.S.
Dentist
Income statement
January 1 to December 31, 19____

Income:

Professional fees	$35,000

Expenses:

Auxiliary salaries	$9,000
Stationery and postage	300
Dental supplies	2,000
Depreciation and amortization	2,000
Office rent	2,000
Professional society expenses	400
Insurance	500
Utilities	700
Waiting room supplies	100
Total expenses	$17,000
Net income	$18,000

Figure 14-9

tal expense of $17,000. If total expenses are subtracted from the professional fees, the difference is profit or net income ($18,000). Note that there is no expense listed for income tax; therefore, the net income is *BIT*, or before income tax.

These income statements can become as complex and as detailed as you want them to be. The question is, "How much is it going to cost, and what benefits will be obtained from purchasing the information?" The primary use of the income statement is to compare it with past income statements to determine any trends and measure progress toward the attainment of financial objectives.

Normally, the objective will be to increase the net income, which can be increased by increasing the income without increasing the expenses-to-income ratio. For example, a 50% overhead for $1,000 results in $500 net income and 50% overhead for $1 million results in a net income of $500,000.

Merely reducing costs or overhead seldom results in quantum leaps in net income, while increasing practice growth and productivity normally results in large changes in net income. The idea of controlling expenses has to be viewed with common sense.

Decreasing expenses does not necessarily bring about good financial management. It normally is far better to increase volume than it is to try to cut costs. If you do want to cut costs, you can generally increase your efficiency by reducing the big items first. There's no use fooling around with reception room supplies at $100. If you could save it all, you wouldn't save much. The places where money can be saved are in the big items, such as salaries. I don't mean to cut the salaries, but rather to use auxiliaries efficiently so that the expense-to-income ratio is reduced. For example, the 1979 figures indicate that the net for a dentist with a hygienist is 43%, and the net without a hygienist is 46%; however, the large increase in professional fees brought in by the hygienist more than makes up for the 3% difference in the overhead.

Ratio Analysis

In a dynamic environment such as exists today with cyclical inflation and stagflation, it is necessary to look at sets of relationships and not at static figures. If someone says that his overhead is good, the question would be, "good compared to what?" For example, if the lab fees increase from $2,000 to $5,000, is that good or bad? The answer is, "compared to what?"

That's where ratio analysis comes into play. There are ratio analyses that monitor relationships between items shown on the balance sheet, those that compare items within the income statement, and still others that compare relationships between items on the income statement and items in the balance sheet. There are also horizontal and vertical ratio analyses. Horizontal analysis compares data horizontally across time. In other words, it compares data from more than one balance sheet or more than one income statement across time. With vertical analysis, all comparisons are made between items on one statement by moving vertically up and down the statement.

Figure 14–10 depicts a form of the income statement called the comparative income statement, designed to facilitate ratio analysis. Two months are depicted. The first column on the right is the previous month and the last column on the left is the present month. The right-hand column indicates that the total fees earned (not necessarily collected) for the previous period were $119,000, of which $26,000 were earned in restorative, $58,000 in crown and bridge, and $35,000 in preventive. The statement also indicates that preventive income was 29% of the total income, crown and bridge was 49%, and restorative was 22%. This is the most basic form of vertical analysis. You now know crown and bridge brings in about twice as much income as the other two areas. Moving to the left, the next column indicates that difference between this month and last month in dollars. Preventive

Professional fees	Amount	%	Var	Amount	%
Preventive	37,000	27	2,000	35,000	29
Crown and bridge	57,000	42	(1,000)	58,000	49
Restorative	43,000	31	17,000	26,000	22
TOTAL FEES	137,000	15	18,000	119,000	
Operating expenses					
Dental supplies	15,000	10.9	5,000	10,000	8.4
Depreciation	6,000	4.4	0	6,000	5.0
Insurance—business	1,500	1.1	0	1,500	1.3
Interest expense	2,400	1.8	0	2,400	2.0
Lab fees	1,500	1.1	700	800	.7
Maintenance and repairs	900	.7	(300)	1,200	1.0
Office expense	5,000	3.6	2,800	2,200	1.8
Salaries	26,000	19.0	5,000	21,000	17.6
Rent	5,600	4.1	0	5,600	4.7
Telephone	3,000	2.2	0	3,000	2.5
Utilities	2,000	1.5	0	2,000	1.7
TOTAL EXPENSES	68,900	50.3	13,200	55,700	46.8

Figure 14–10 Comparative income statement

income increased $2,000, crown and bridge decreased $1,000 (notice that the parentheses are for negative income), and restorative income increased $17,000, for a total of $43,000.

A comparison and evaluation of the new percentages is an example of horizontal analysis. Preventive income as a percentage of total income has decreased by 2%, crown and bridge dropped 7%, and restorative went up 9% so that crown and bridge no longer dominated the practice. The total fees were $137,000 or a gain in income of 15% over the previous month.

It is possible to do both horizontal and vertical analysis by comparing one month with the other or by going up and down the columns within a month. For example, dental supplies have increased from $5,000 to $15,000, now being 10.9% of gross income. Here ratios are established between gross income and operating expenses. Now, the 10.9% might not look like much, but if you work it out on your calculator, you will see that cost of supplies went up 29% (10.9 ÷ 8.4) while total income went up only 15%. If they had gone up at the same rate, then supplies would still be at 8.4% of gross income.

These are the kinds of changes you must look into if the practice is to be efficient. In the case of a fixed cost such as depreciation, you can see that as the fixed cost stays constant, if the income increases, then the percentage of depreciation or the ratio of depreciation to total income begins to drop. It dropped from 1.3 to 1.1%, a drop of 14%, which is exactly reflected by the change in income. The same situation exists with the business insurance and interest expense.

Lab fees went up from $800 to $1,500, an increase of $700 which is a 57% (1.1% ÷ .7%) increase over the previous month. This should be cause for concern, since the bulk of the lab fees should be tied to the crown and bridge operation, which actually decreased over the time period. You can also see at the bottom of the chart that the ratio of total expenses to total earnings was 50.3% this month and 46.8% last month, which is an increase of 7% in overhead but an increase of 15% in fees earned. This is a very favorable trend in that production increased without a comparable increase in overhead.

Here are some examples of commonly used key ratios. Probably one of the best known ratios is the *current ratio,* or the ratio of current assets to current liabilities, which indicates your ability to pay debts. Referring back to Figure 14–1 (the balance sheet), the current ratio is equal to $51,000 (current assets) divided by $11,000 (current liabilities) or a ratio of 4.6 to 1. If the practice were to close as of now, you would be able to pay off the short-term liabilities since you have $4.60 worth of current assets for every $1.00 of current debt.

Another important ratio is *working capital turnover,* which is gross income divided by the working capital and is a measure of efficiency. You have to go to two different places to get the information; the comparative income statement provides the gross income ($137,000), and the balance sheet provides the working capital, which is current assets minus current liabilities ($51,000 − $11,000, or $40,000). Dividing $137,000 by $40,000 indicates a turnover rate of 3.4%. When the rate is too low, it shows an inefficient use of assets. When it is too high, it indicates a vulnerability to creditors because of an insufficient amount of working capital on hand.

The *average collection period* is an important ratio. To derive this ratio, divide the credit sales for the period by the days in the period. The result equals the average daily credit for the period. Then, divide the total accounts receivable by the average daily credit sales to arrive at the number of days money was tied up in accounts receivable. For example, if $150,000 of credit has been extended in a six-month period using 20 working days per month, there would be 120 days in the period, which would result in $1,250 as the average amount of daily credit sales. Now, assume $80,000 in accounts receivable as the average accounts receivable for the last six months. Dividing $80,000 by $1,250 results in 64 days as the average collection period, which is an indication of the effectiveness of your collection policies.

The next ratio of interest is known as *R.O.I.,* or *return on investment.* The numerator is net income from the income statement, and the denominator is capital employed, which is total assets from the balance sheet. In this case, you have income ($137,000) minus expenses ($68,900), which equals net income before taxes ($68,100). To get the capital employed, go back to the balance sheet to find current assets ($40,000) plus fixed assets ($60,000), which equals total assets or capital invested ($100,000). Dividing $68,100 in the numerator by $100,000 in the denominator results in a return of 68%.

Another important ratio is that of *accounts receivable to gross income,* which should not exceed 17% or 2 months under the present economic conditions. The current assets portion of the balance sheet provides the accounts receivable ($35,000), and gross income ($137,000) is provided by the comparative income statement. Dividing $35,000 by $137,000 provides a ratio of 25.5%, which is a little higher than recommended.

Cash Flow Budgeting

Now let's move on to *cash flow budgeting,* or the control of working capital. Recall from the balance sheet that the working capital was equal to current assets minus current liabilities. At first glance, it appears that the higher the current assets, the better, but this is not the case. If it becomes too high, there is the problem of a loss of investment opportunities if the money is sitting in a bank account earning either no interest or a very minimal amount. Excess cash should be put into investments which will realize the maximum return consistent with the degree of risk that you're willing to take.

If, on the other hand, current assets gets too low, you will be unable to pay your bills. In this case, if no other action is taken, your credit rating will get to the point where you'll be unable to purchase the things that you need or pay your staff and the practice will go bankrupt.

A situation that's almost as bad is a continual scramble at the last minute to find money to pay current expenses, which will require acceptance of less than the best deal available on a loan. When seeking a loan, you must shop for money just as you would shop for any other commodity if you wish to buy at the lowest price.

It is important also to be very realistic about accounts receivable and their effect on control of working capital. If working capital consisted only of accounts receivable and no cash, it would be a pretty risky situation, requiring drastic action to cash in on those accounts receivable at the earliest possible moment to meet the monthly liabilities.

If you do decide that you need a loan — and it's not a bad thing at times to have to borrow money to run a business — you must be prepared to present your case in a manner which will guarantee acceptance by loan officers of banks. Loan officers will be reluctant to grant money if they can't be shown (1) how much is needed, and (2) when it can be repaid.

It is important to realize that profits are not the same as cash. Cash in current assets can be way up, but so can liabilities. It's the difference between the two that spells success or failure. For example, too often in the past, building contractors were making bids on construction providing a 10% profit, and then borrowing money at 12% to 13%. While they were doing a tremendous business with high cash flows and cash on hand, they didn't realize that at the same time the long-term liabilities were increasing even faster. So the faster they worked, the more they lost.

Cash flow budgeting is a very simple process of determining the cash on hand at the beginning of the month, estimating monthly income and adding the two together to get a cash balance. Then expenses for the month are determined and subtracted from the cash balance to obtain the ending balance or cash on hand at the end of the month. If it's negative, you're in trouble and will need to do something about it. Figure 14–11 illustrates cash flow budgeting.

In the first month, you estimated an income of $1,100 in cash, and zero accounts receivable. (Note that accounts receivable [A/R] were earned, but that none would be collected until the next month.) Accounts receivable as such are not included in the budget — only an estimate of the amount of A/R that will be collected. The total income for the month is $1,100, and an estimate of operating and living expenses was $7,225. The difference in parentheses (parentheses are used to indicate negative figures) is the cash balance at the end of the first month, −$6,125.

You estimated that business was going to pick up in the second month with $3,055 of cash income and collections of $440 from last month's A/Rs for a total income of $3,495. The cash on hand at the beginning of the month is −$6,125 plus an estimated $7,031 in expenses equals a negative cash balance at the end of the month of $9,661. Moving into the third month, you forecasted a collection of $2,887 in cash and that the accounts receivable would really begin to flow in at $1,960, for a total income of $4,847. The cash on hand now has grown to −$9,661 with an estimated disbursement of $7,081 or almost $17,000 from which we subtract the $4,847 income for a negative balance of $11,895. In the fourth month, the forecast is for $3,520

Use the following parameters to estimate loan required for first six months of practice.

Month	1	2	3	4
Fees cash	1,100	3,055	2,887	3,520
Collect A/R	-0-	440	1,960	2,100
Total receipts	1,100	3,495	4,847	5,620
Cash on hand	-0-	(6,125)	(9,661)	(11,895)
Estimated disbursement	7,225	7,031	7,081	7,231
Estimated cash balance End of month	(6,125)	(9,661)	(11,895)	(13,506)
Revised — 18,000 loan				
Fees cash	1,100	3,055	2,887	3,520
Collect A/R	-0-	440	1,960	2,100
Total receipts	1,100	3,495	4,847	5,620
Cash on hand beg.	18,000	11,875	8,339	6,105
Estimated disbursement	7,225	7,031	7,081	7,231
Estimated cash balance	11,875	8,339	5,005	4,494

Figure 14–11   Cash flow budget

in cash receipts plus $2,100 from receivables for a total of $5,620. Applying that against our −$11,895 cash on hand, and an estimated expense of $7,231, which is almost $19,000, and subtracting the $5,620, results in a −$13,506 cash flow at the end of the fourth month. Obviously, if nothing was done, the practice would go broke.

So, what can you do? You estimate a need for $18,000 which should more than cover your expenses and take care of any miscalculations, keeping in mind that interest is not payable until the money is actually withdrawn from the bank. The bottom of Figure 14–11 depicts the effect of the loan on the cash flow. At the beginning of the first month, cash on hand was $18,000, and at the end of the month, it was $11,875. Working on through the months, applying the same figures as before, we end up at the end of the fourth month with $4,494. The cash flow into the practice has been showing a steady increase of about $800–$1,000/month, and a continuation of the forecast would indicate that a negative cash flow could be avoided, and as income continued to increase, a reasonable dissolution of the loan could be made. That is in essence the budgeting process for the control of cash flow. Having performed the calculations in Figure 14–11, you are in a good position to convince the bank loan officer that you are a businessman with a well-planned program who should be granted a loan.

Breakeven Analysis

Now let us consider the breakeven analyses. To do so, we must first review some terminology so as to grasp the concept.

Fixed Expenses are those expenses that do not vary in the short run with the amount of dentistry performed, but rather are based on the passage of time. Some accountants refer to fixed costs as *time costs.* These can include items such as rent, utilities, and insurance. In other words, it costs a certain amount just to run the office even if there are no patients.

Variable Expenses are those expenses that occur only as a result of patient treatment, such as laboratory fees, dental supplies, drugs, and bad debts.

Overhead is another word for expenses, and is usually referred to as a percent of the gross income. Total overhead = variable expense plus fixed expense.

Variable Expense Ratio is the ratio of variable expenses to total practice income. This percentage normally will not change as the total practice revenue changes. For example, if your practice had a variable expense ratio of 20 percent when your gross was $90,000, it would normally be approximately 20 percent if your gross increased to $150,000. The variable expense ratio would change, however, if the ratio of crown and bridge to all other procedures changed because of the change in laboratory fees.

Breakeven Point is the point at which your gross income exactly equals all expenses.

Figure 14-12 compares the traditional income statement at the top of the figure with an income statement prepared using the fixed and variable expense concept.

Figure 14-13 is the classic breakeven diagram with dollars on the vertical axis and units of production on the horizontal axis. The fixed costs, which do not vary with production, are shown as a horizontal line. The variable costs, which are only incurred with production, are represented by a line starting at the intersection of the vertical axis and the horizontal line of the fixed costs and extending up to the right. The difference between the variable cost line and the horizontal axis represents the total cost for producing that many units. The difference between the variable cost line and the fixed cost line represents the variable cost of producing that many units.

Income statement assuming $150,000 gross income
(data provided by Healthco)

PRACTICE INCOME		$150,000
Rent		6,345
Utilities		2,430
Salaries		29,580
Insurance		1,440
Depreciation		4,005
Professional liability		765
Interest		1,440
Repairs		900
Legal		990
Travel		2,190
Miscellaneous		4,425
Laboratory		17,610
Drugs		480
Dental supplies		9,000
Bad debts		2,655
	TOTAL	84,255
	NET INCOME	$65,745

Income statement using fixed and variable cost categories

Gross income		$150,000
Less variable expenses		
Laboratory fees		17,610
Drugs		480
Dental supplies		9,000
Bad debts		2,625
	TOTAL VARIABLE COST	$29,745
Less fixed expenses		
Rent		6,345
Utilities		2,430
Salaries		29,580
Insurance		1,440
Depreciation		4,005
Professional liability		765
Interest		1,440
Repairs		900
Legal		990
Travel		2,190
Miscellaneous		4,425
	TOTAL FIXED COST	$54,510
	TOTAL	$84,255
	NET INCOME	$65,745

Figure 14-12

You also plot the net income received for the number of units produced. You can see that until the income line crosses the variable cost line, net income is negative or the practice is operating at a loss. Where the income line and the total expense line cross is the point at which the income exactly equals expenses (fixed plus variable), or the breakeven point. If the lines never cross, the practice will go bankrupt, which is why breakeven analysis is so important in fee-setting. If the gross income line climbs above the variable expense line, the vertical distance between the two lines is net income. To review: there are variable costs, fixed costs, gross income, and the breakeven point at which the income exactly equals variable costs plus fixed costs.

There is another way of doing this that might make a little more sense to us in dentistry, since we don't normally deal in homogeneous units. Figure 14-14 has dollars on the vertical axis and time on the horizontal axis. The following example will illustrate the use of this technique to determine the breakeven point in the first year of a practice. In that one year, it is estimated that $60,000 worth of fixed costs will accumulate. A line is drawn from 0 dollars at the bottom left ascending at an angle to reach $60,000 at the end of the year. It is also estimated that there will be $25,510 of variable costs, and a slightly curved line is drawn because this variable cost increases at a different rate, as predicted in Figure 14-15. The predicted income was based on the estimated percent of patient contact time per hour that the practice was open, which was called *utilization.* For the first two months, a 30% utilization was estimated, 50% for the next two, 60% for the next two, and then leveling off at 80% of the dentist time spent in patient contact for the remainder of the year. Below % utilization you can see the number of *productive hours* available. If the estimates are accurate, breakeven would occur in about the ninth month.

If the total overhead of $85,500 is divided by the hours available (1,216), we would find that the overhead equals $70 per hour, and that to break even, it would be necessary to earn $70 per hour. Looking at the variable costs per hour, we find that it's $25,520 divided by 1,216, or $21 per hour.

Here we introduce the idea of *contribution to margin.* If the $21 per hour variable cost is subtracted from the $70 per hour fee, we would have a contribution to margin of $49 per hour using the formula that total overhead = fixed cost + variable cost, or that fixed cost = total cost − variable cost.

It is possible to compute the breakeven mathematically by dividing the fixed cost of $60,000 by the $49 which is the contribution to margin. In other words, the contribution to margin is equal to the total fee less the variable cost. The remainder of the fee is available to absorb the fixed cost. In this manner, we estimate 1,224 hours of patient contact to breakeven

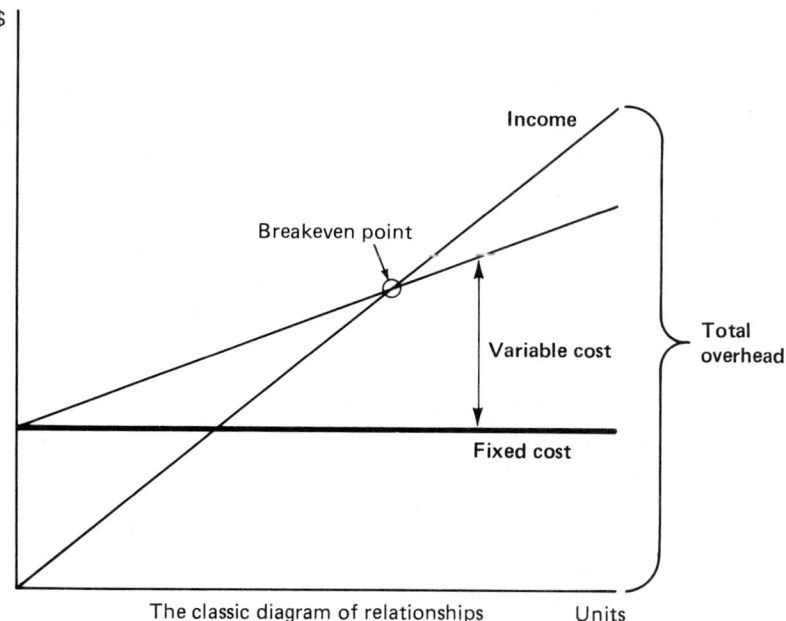

Figure 14-13 Breakeven analysis

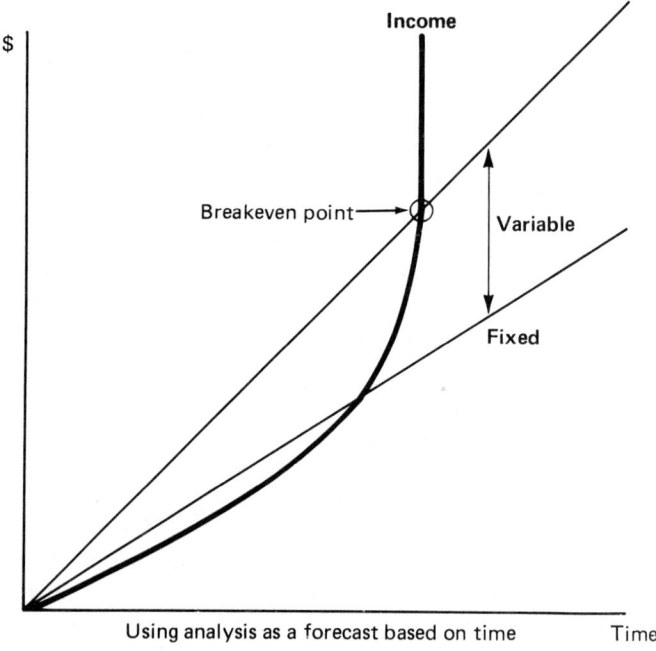

Figure 14-14 Breakeven analysis

	1	2	3	4	5	6	7	8	9	10	11	12
Fixed costs:												
Loan	700	---	---	---	---	---	---	---	---	---	---	---
Rent	600	---	---	---	---	---	---	---	---	---	---	---
Insurance	100	---	---	---	---	---	---	---	---	---	---	---
Telephone	100	---	---	---	---	---	---	---	---	---	---	---
Utilities	300	---	---	---	---	---	---	---	---	---	---	---
Salaries	3,000	---	---	---	---	---	---	---	---	---	---	---
TOTAL	5,000	10,000	15,000	20,000	25,000	30,000	35,000	40,000	45,000	50,000	55,000	60,000
Variable costs:												
Supplies	100	150	---	---	---	180	---	200	---	250	300	---
Salaries	1,000	---	---	1,400	---	1,500	---	---	---	---	1,550	---
Lab fees	150	200	250	300	400	500	600	700	800	900	1,000	---
TOTAL	1,250	2,600	4,000	5,850	7,800	9,980	12,260	14,460	17,160	19,810	22,660	25,510
Overhead	6,200	12,600	19,000	25,900	32,800	40,000	47,300	54,500	62,200	69,800	77,700	85,500
% Utilization	30	---	50	---	60	---	80	---	---	---	---	---
Productive hours	48	---	80	---	96	---	128	---	---	---	---	---
Cumulative Based upon $160/month	48	96	176	256	352	448	576	704	832	960	1,088	1,216

Figure 14–15 Breakeven forecast

which is very, very close to the computation arrived at in a more complex manner.

A still better way to compute the breakeven point is with the following formula.

$$\text{Breakeven} = \frac{\text{fixed expense} + \text{desired net income}}{(1 - \text{variable expense ratio})}$$

You will recall that this formula was used and discussed in Chapter 4, The Associateship.

Another important form of analysis is *non-financial analysis*, which focuses mainly on patient care and staff effectiveness, concerning itself with such things as quality assurance. For example, the number of redos — evaluating those instances in which there was poor case selection or improper techniques, or poor choices of materials. Both financial and medical records should be systematically reviewed to insure neatness, accuracy and completeness. Patients' complaints should be analyzed for patterns indicating insensitivity to patient needs.

From the standpoint of preventive dentistry, if you're really preventive-oriented, have plaque indexes been established for the patients, and are they getting better, staying the same, or getting worse? If so, why? Looking at practice growth, how many patients have been lost and gained in the last year? How about referrals? Who's doing the referrals? How many of them? What's the trend — are the referrals increasing or decreasing? And why?

Other items are production and resource utilization. The resource utilization really ties into the patient contact. How much time is actually spent in patient contact? There is your time, the time of the staff, and the time of the patients to consider. Are the operatories being fully utilized? What is a reasonable figure for such utilization? These are the kinds of things that the effective dentist must know. How much time is spent in operative, in periodontics, in endodontics? Look at how the percentage of time spent in these areas compared with the percentage of fees earned. It's a good way to get a better feel for the rationale of the fee schedule.

Waiting time is particularly important. Wasting the time of your patients is a good way to lose them. Appointment scheduling should be evaluated by analyzing the waiting time per appointment, including the waiting time in the reception area and the actual versus scheduled time used. If an emergency period has been designated, what percentage of these emergency periods is actually being utilized? And lastly, what is the effectiveness of the recall system?

Summary

Conducting recurring financial analyses is essential to operating an effective dental practice. Financial analysis requires the support of a good office recordkeeping system for its data. The tools of financial analysis are the balance sheet with its recording of assets and liabilities; the income statement with its gross income, expenses and net income; the ratio analysis which permits controlling for changes; the cash flow budget which permits an evaluation of the availability of cash for future operations, and the breakeven analysis which provides forecast information upon which to estimate your ability to make a profit.

Review Questions

1. List and define the elements of the balance sheet.
2. Discuss the elements that make up the overhead of a practice and discuss how these elements react with changes in production.
3. Construct a breakeven chart showing the following: fixed expense, variable expense, gross income, and breakeven point.
4. Given the following data, determine the breakeven point.
   fixed expense = $60,000
   desired net income = $80,000
   variable expense ratio = .20

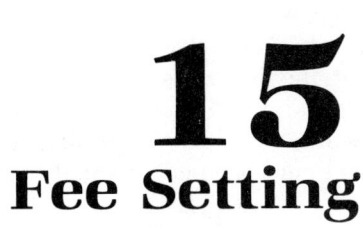

15
Fee Setting

Learning Objectives

Upon completion of this chapter, you should be able to:

- Discuss the factors which affect the fee-setting process.
- Compute a fee for a procedure given the income statement and the operatory hours of the practice.

Introduction

In Chapter 14 we discussed financial analysis. In this chapter we are going to discuss how financial analysis can contribute to the fee-setting process.

Fee setting is vital to the survival of the practice. While some dentists may feel that a concern with fee setting and the financial aspects of the practice is somehow unprofessional, unless the fee-setting process provides the practice with enough money to stay in business, you cannot meet your responsibilities to the patients, the dental staff, or to your family. Fees must provide for modern equipment and for the salaries of a skilled and motivated staff.

In general, the causes for an inadequate fee schedule are:

- A general lack of business knowledge, which results in a lack of the complete and accurate financial records which are necessary for computing the costs of running the practice.
- A lack of the incentive to accomplish adequate financial analysis.

These two factors can lead to a lack of confidence in dealing both with other dentists and with the patients on business matters.

While fee setting is an important element in dental practice management, the process is fairly complex and not fully understood by many practitioners. A 1979 survey indicated that 60 percent of the dentists polled based their fees on what other dentists charged.

Others have commented that the reason many dentists are defensive about discussing fees with their patients is because they have not been able to develop a rational system in their own minds for defending their fees. Still others have been more harsh in their comments, stating that the ADA should encourage a time-based schedule rather than a fee-for-service schedule because it has been known for many years that the fee schedule in dentistry is irrational.

There are basically three ways to set fees:

1. according to the cost of services
2. according to demand
3. according to the competition

The last two ways of setting fees will not be discussed in this book. We will discuss the procedures involved in setting fees based upon cost of services.

Some have asked why we don't set standard fees as some consumer advocate groups are recommending. The standard fee does not appear to be an adequate approach for a number of reasons. First, despite best intentions, and as attested to by the need for peer review, the quality of services rendered varies from dentist to dentist. If we believe in the free enterprise system, those who have developed skills above those of their contemporaries should be able to command a higher fee.

Similarly, those who have attempted to increase the quality of dental care by investing in the latest equipment and training must also be permitted to recoup the cost of that equipment. It is also apparent that the location has an effect on the fee schedule. The cost of living in New York City is far higher than in Lafayette County, Florida. To charge the residents of Lafayette County on the same fee schedule as those in New York would result in denying adequate dental care to the poorer segment of society.

While it cannot be denied that the actions of the competition will have an important effect upon fee setting, it should not be the sole basis for determining fees. This will be discussed further at a later point in this section.

The Steps in Fee Setting

The following are the steps in setting fees based upon costs of services rendered.

Step 1 Figure 15-1 is an example of the process used to determine the number of hours per year that you will be in patient contact. Patient contact is the number of hours you are actually treating a patient. This can vary considerably from available dentist time. The first part of the computation in Figure 15-1 derives the time available by subtracting from 365 days those days that will not be available for treating patients, i.e., days set aside for vacations, holidays, and continuing education. In this particular

```
Maximum days              365
Holidays                 −  7
                          358
Sundays                  − 52
                          306
One other day off        − 52
                          254
Vacation                 − 14
                          240
Meetings, illness, etc.  − 10
                          230 × 8 = 1,840
Patient contact %         × .80
                          184 × 8 hours = 1,472 hours
```

Figure 15-1 Computation of annual patient contact time

example, the remaining time available for patient treatment was 230 days for the year.

However, even the most efficient dentist cannot maintain a 100 percent utilization of his time by being in patient contact. Time must be allowed for administration, case studies, and operatory set-up. In addition, in the case of a new practice or in times of recession, the patient flow may be insufficient to fill all the available treatment time. Deciding on the percentage of time that the dentist will be in patient contact is a judgment call that must be based either upon experience or your best judgment.

In either case, the decision is not irrevocable. The available time and the fees based upon the estimates may be adjusted as necessary to allow for the many factors that may change. In this case, an 80 percent patient contact factor was applied, reducing the number of available days from 230 to 184. Multiplying the number of days by the number of hours the dentist intends to operate each day (in this case 8 hours) results in a total of 1,472 hours being available for the year. The same result can be obtained by multiplying the 8 hours by percent utilization (8 × .8 = 6.4), and then multiplying 6.4 hours by 230 days.

Step 2 Figure 15–2 presents a hypothetical example of the costs of the dental practice for the year in question. The actual cost of operating the practice is shown as $52,263. Note that a *withdrawal* is indicated immediately under that amount. This is entered to demonstrate that your desired net income is to be considered as part of the cost of dental care delivery.

In this case, we assumed a net income of $20,000 before taxes. If desired, it is also possible to include your estimated taxes as a portion of the cost of operating the practice. Here also, we come to one of the reasons that standardized fee schedules are not adequate. Each dentist must decide what aspirations he will have concerning his standard of living.

At the bottom of Figure 15–2, the computations are shown demonstrating how to combine the information in Figures 15–1 and 15–2 to produce a desired cost per unit of time. This is obtained by dividing total costs by the estimated number of hours in patient contact. The results indicate $392.00 per day, $49.00 per hour, $.82 per minute as the minimum requirement to break even.

Step 3 Figure 15–3 is an example of how to translate cost per unit of time into fees per procedure. For example, the fee for a one-surface amalgam is computed by first determining the variable cost for the procedure — in this case, the cost of the rubber dam, anesthesia, bib, and a spill of amalgam. Note that in the listing of expenses, variable costs were

2 Aux's salaries with salary tax (2 × $9,880)	$19,760
Receptionist	9,880
Rent	4,024
Utilities	2,000
Insurance	1,000
Depreciation	2,544
Liability	500
Interest payments	1,000
Repairs	570
Legal/professional fees	635
Fees — C.E., etc.	1,000
Drugs	350
General supplies	5,000
Bad debts	1,000
Miscellaneous	3,000
	$52,263
Withdrawal	20,000
TOTAL	$72,263

72,263/1,472 = $49/hour
$49/hour/60 = .82/minute
$49 × 8 hours = $392/day
$392 × 20 days = $7,840

Allowance for risk (redos, adjustments)

Figure 15–2 Annual fixed cost

Assumption: Meet fixed cost of $49/hour ($.82/minute)
  Variable cost = $.39 for rubber dam, anesthesia, bib
       $.82/spill of amalgam
  Time/surface = 30'
  Prep time/patient = 10'

1 Surface amalgam = 10' + 30' = 40' × $.82 = $33 for time
       + .39 + .82 variable cost = $33 + $1 = $34
2 Surface amalgam = 10' + 30' + 30' = 70' × $.82 = $57
       + .39 + 4 × .82 = $4 = $61
3 Surface amalgam = 10' + 3 × 30' = 100' × $.82 = $82
       + .39 + 6 × .82 = $5 + $82 = $87

Figure 15–3 Computing operative fees

190 FEE SETTING

not listed, i.e., laboratory fees and dental supplies. The reason for this will become evident as we proceed.

You estimate that it will take 10 minutes to greet and seat the patient, administer the anesthesia, and install the rubber dam, after which you will take 30 minutes to prepare, condense and carve the restoration. Multiplying the time for the procedure by the cost per minute ($.82) results in $33.00 for the time plus $1.00 for the materials, giving a total fee of $34.00 for a one-surface amalgam. Similar examples are shown for a two- and a three-surface amalgam.

Testing the Fee Using Breakeven Analysis

Step 4 You can test the feasibility of your fee schedule by seeing if you have the capability to break even in a given time period. Figure 15-4 demonstrates how to use time absorption techniques to compute a breakeven point. The basis of the time absorption approach is that fixed costs are time costs. As discussed previously, fixed costs do not vary with production, but do add up as time passes. In this case, whether you treat patients or not, you must pay $.82 per minute, $49.00 per hour, and $392.00 a day for the practice. It is then incumbent upon you and your staff to produce enough income to absorb the fixed cost.

In the example, the formula for breakeven volume is fixed cost divided by the fee minus the variable cost. In the case of the example for the two-surface amalgam in Figure 15-4, the fee is $61.00, from which the $4.00 variable cost is subtracted. The fixed cost of $392.00 per day is then divided by $57.00 to determine that 7 two-surface amalgams must be produced per day to break even. Our time for accomplishing a two-surface amalgam is estimated at 70 minutes, and multiplying by the seven required to break even, we see that we can just exactly break even in an eight-hour day.

Many practitioners would be well advised to review this exercise and apply it to the examination of their existing fees to see if some of those procedures are not paying for themselves. If not, serious consideration should be given to either improving the operating procedure to reduce time and variable cost, or failing that, to consider referring those procedures to other dentists who for various reasons are able to break even on those procedures.

Fixed cost/day = $528.00

Example: Breakeven volume = $\dfrac{\text{Fixed cost}}{\text{Fee} - \text{variable cost}}$

2-Surface amalgam: Fee = $61, variable cost = $4

Breakeven for a day = $\dfrac{\$392}{\$61 - \$4}$ = 7 two-surface amalgams/day

Check for capability   7 × 70′ = 490′ = 8 hours

3-Surface amalgam: Fee = $87, variable cost = $5

For a day = $\dfrac{\$392}{\$87 - \$5}$ = 5/day

Check for capability   5 × 100′ = 500′ = 8 hours

Figure 15-4 Computing breakeven using time absorption or contribution to margin (on a daily basis)

What we have discussed in this section is an approach to the problem of fee setting. While this procedure does provide you with a *base line*, or the minimum you can charge without losing money, other additional factors still remain to be considered.

You must consider the risk of the procedure in the form of redos and additional visits, i.e., such items as fractured amalgams and adjustments of removable prosthodontics. Equally important is the consideration of what the competition is charging for similar procedures. If the fees of the other dentists in the area are significantly lower, it is possible that your practice either has serious problems in efficiency and utilization of resources, or that the other dentists are in serious trouble because they have failed to adjust fees to keep pace with the ever increasing operating costs.

The problem will also arise of what to do for the patients who cannot afford the treatment they need. There are at least two possible solutions. One is to set aside a certain portion of your time to provide for the needy dental patient and keep track of your use of that time. This will provide a logical and defensible way of drawing the line beyond which the donation of additional time would jeopardize the success of the practice.

As is sometimes the case, it is easier to deny additional care to members of the same family by explaining that the practice can only afford to provide a certain amount of free dental care, or care at a reduced price, and that providing additional care for the family will deny it to other needy patients.

Summary

Fee setting based on cost data and time per procedure will provide you with the minimum fee for a procedure that will prevent you from losing money. The fees must be derived by keeping accurate data on costs and time required for each procedure. This will still not completely answer the problem of setting fees, for you must still estimate the risk factor and compare each procedure in the treatment plan against a hypothetical average procedure and adjust the fee accordingly. Once this is done, you must compare your fee schedule with the fees charged by other dentists in your area and adjust as necessary.

Review Questions

1. Compute the breakeven cost per hour given a practice that is closed for three weeks a year plus an additional 10 holidays, and which has a 60 percent dentist utilization rate. The fixed overhead is estimated at $100,000, the variable expenses at $30,000, and the desired net is $150,000.
2. Given the above data, compute the fee for a procedure which takes 45 minutes to accomplish.
3. Given the data in questions 2 and 3, plus the fact that the variable cost of the procedure accomplished in question 2 is $5.00, compute the number of these procedures required to break even in one day.

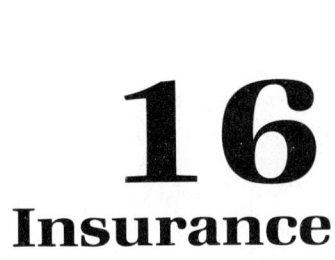

16
Insurance

Learning Objectives

Upon completion of this chapter, you should be able to:

- Discuss the factors to be considered when setting up a comprehensive risk management program to include life, disability, medical, and overhead insurance.
- Explain the purpose of the buy-sell agreement.

Introduction

There are various types of insurance policies that will be required for your practice:

- Those that will protect your earning potential (life, health and disability insurance).

- Those that will protect you from claims by others (liability).
- Those that will protect your property.

Another way to look at insurance is as risk management. There are certain risks that everyone faces both in leading their daily life and in conducting a business or dental practice. The way that you can reduce the amount of risk that you face is to share this risk with an insurance company by purchasing one of their policies.

Protection of Earning Potential

Life insurance is in reality an attempt to protect against the risk of losing your earning potential. The reason that you need to protect your earning potential is to provide for those who depend on you for their support. In the early years, the dependence upon your support is more likely to be minimal. For example, a single person may not have any person to support. Upon marriage, if the spouse is capable of earning a living, the amount of protection required is still minimal. As children are born into the family, the demand for protection of the earning potential necessarily increases for it would be very difficult for a spouse to earn a suitable living and raise children at the same time.

In the early years of your career, the availability of resources is likely to limit the amount of money available for insurance, so it is important to obtain maximum coverage at minimum cost. While it is sometimes sentimental to buy large policies when you marry, it is wise to recall that the earning potential of a spouse without children is pretty good, and it is even better if the spouse has been trained for a profession.

So, prior to buying insurance of any kind, you must be able to answer three questions: (1) Why do I want to buy it? (2) How much should I buy? and (3) When should I buy?

In answer to the question of why you should buy insurance, since some of you will be seeking loans for starting your practice, associateship or other practice mode, you will find that insurance coverage for the loan will be required by the lender. Also, if you enter into a partnership, you will be involved in a *buy-sell* agreement, which we discussed in Chapter 4. Another reason for buying the insurance we have already discussed is to protect those who will depend upon you for income.

In answer to the question of how much to buy, we are faced with a personal decision of how much to sacrifice now to provide for the future. This decision is complicated by the life style that you and your dependents desire, but as a minimum, the coverage should be enough to pay the outstanding debts in the event of your death. Beyond that bare minimum, you can compute your family's living expense requirements and subtract your assets now available. The difference is the amount of insurance that would be required to maintain their present standard of living without your income.

As for when to buy insurance, you must consider the following:

1. In time to provide the security for loans as required by the lender.
2. When you have a family which would detract from the ability of your spouse to raise the children and work at the same time in the event of your death.
3. To provide for your insurability.

Most insurance companies will provide you with a policy early in life which guarantees that you may always purchase additional insurance as desired without a physical examination. If you do not protect your insurability at an early age, you may find that as you age, insurance will not be available due to your failing health.

You must carefully read any life insurance policy to make sure that provisions for future insurability are included. This is particularly true in times of inflation. A life insurance program that was considered more than adequate ten years ago is submarginal now and requires the purchase of additional insurance. If insurability were not guaranteed, buying additional insurance might not be possible, or might only be possible at a very high fee.

The basis of the buy-sell agreement is a life insurance policy. The buy-sell agreement is an important feature of risk management in multi-dentist practices such as groups, partnerships and associateships. Normally, this agreement is applicable when more than one dentist has an interest in the survival of the business after the death of one of the owners.

The purpose of the buy-sell agreement is to provide a quick and legal means for the other owners of the business to assume full control of the business upon the death of one of the owners.

For illustration, we will explain the use of the buy-sell agreement in a partnership. If one of the partners in a practice should die, his share of the practice would pass to his legal heir(s). The surviving partner then is subject to the will of the heir(s), who may wish to sell their share to the survivor, or to the highest bidder. It is not unusual for the practice to be closed while the case goes through litigation which could take years, at the end of which time the practice would be worthless. Even if this situation were somehow avoided, there is still the problem of determining the value of the deceased partner's share of the practice for sale and tax purposes. The IRS has been known to assess a value far in excess of other estimates.

To avoid these problems, it is possible to execute the buy-sell agreement in which the partners agree upon a fair price for their share of the practice and then purchase life insurance policies which will pay that amount on the death of one of the partners. Normally, when such an agreement is made and funded as described, the deceased dentist's share of the practice will immediately pass to the survivor without undue delay. Further, if the agreement has been drawn up properly, the IRS will accept the value of the practice as stipulated in the agreement, the heirs will receive a fair price for their share of the practice, the surviving partner will be able to deduct the proper amount of the price from his taxes, and there is far less chance of the practice being tied up in litigation.

Types of Life Insurance

The three primary types of life insurance are *cash value, endowment,* and *term.* In the case of the cash value, as premiums are paid the cash value increases, and the amount of insurance actually provided for by the company decreases so that both together will equal the face value of the policy. The advantage of a cash value policy is that it is possible to borrow against the cash value at rates considerably below the going market rate. Both cash value and term insurance can be used as collateral for a loan. The *limited pay life policy* is a policy in which the buyer pays for a specified number of years. This also has a cash value, but the premiums are usually much higher.

Another type of policy is the endowment policy, which either pays at death or after a specified number of years if you survive. This is a very high premium policy because you are paying the insurance company to save your money for you.

The best buy in insurance is term insurance, which may be either renewable or non-renewable. Again, remember the previous discussion on insurability. Term insurance is issued for a stated period of time, say from three to five years, and must be renewed at the end of each period at a higher premium as you age. This is the cheapest insurance that can be purchased and provides the maximum amount of coverage with the minimum amount of cash.

There are a number of important features that you should check for in a life insurance policy. Among them is the provision to waive the premiums in the event of your total disability. You might also want to consider double indemnity, which pays double in the case of accidental death. But the most important feature is the guaranteed insurance clause, which states that you may purchase more insurance at a later date.

Before leaving the subject of life insurance, I think it is important to emphasize the difference between insurance which is a risk management device, and investments. While under some unusual circumstances, life insurance can possibly be conceived of as an investment, in general the return on life insurance cannot match the return on other types of investments such as stocks, bonds and real estate. In the long run, you will normally be better off financially to buy term insurance rather than the other more expensive types of policies and to invest the difference in one of the true investment programs just mentioned.

Disability Insurance

Another consideration in the protection of your income which is particularly applicable to the dentist is that of disability insurance. Disability is generally more serious with dentists than for the average person because the dental practice depends primarily upon your ability to produce the income. When a dentist is disabled, the income drops immediately.

Generally, after you have been disabled for 90 days the practice will begin to lose patients rapidly, and statistics indicate that between the ages of 25 and 65, 70% of the people will be disabled for 90 days, and 30% will be disabled for six months.

There are a number of types of disability insurance. There is the *noncancellable,* which is guaranteed renewable and also the most expensive. There is a *guaranteed renewable* which cannot be cancelled, but can increase premiums; this is the second most expensive. There is also a *group insurance* which will be available to you as a dentist through the ADA or the state dental association. It is usually renewable as long as a master contract is in force, and normally, you can increase the premiums based upon experience.

In examining your policy, the definition of disability is critical. The best definition is *the inability to perform the functions of one's regular profession.* This definition can be particularly important for a specialist. If the policy stated *the inability to perform dentistry,* then it might not cover you if you were a specialist and were disabled but were still capable of conducting a general practice.

Also, it is important to know how long the policy pays. Policies may pay for short-term (two to five years) or long-term (to age 65). If you choose the short-term policy, you face the chance of being uninsurable later on as a result of incurring the disability in the first place; so be sure to check the benefit period and also the waiting period. The longer the wait between the occurrence of disability and the start of payments, the cheaper the insurance. However, it requires that you be able to self-insure for the waiting period. This includes the salaries and overhead for your staff as well as for your own family.

Certain tax implications are involved. It is highly recommended that you review the provisions and the implications of all insurance policies with a certified public accountant. In general, in a solo practice, the premiums are not deductible, but the payoff is tax exempt. In the case of an incorporated practice, if the premiums are paid by the corporation, they are deductible to the corporation but the payoff to you is taxable, so allow for this in the coverage.

In other words, if you pay for the insurance from your own pocket, it is normally true that the payoff is non-taxable. If someone else buys it for you, then it is taxable, and you must allow for this in your estate planning for the amount of insurance you require.

The difference between a non-cancellable policy and a guaranteed renewable is that a non-cancellable policy cannot be cancelled nor can the agreed-upon premium be changed until the specified age has been reached (normally 65). A guaranteed renewable policy guarantees that the policy may be renewed, but makes no commitment as to the premium which normally will increase with age or if your physical condition deteriorates.

You should also consider the problem of keeping the practice going in the event of your disability. *Office overhead insurance* is available, which is different from providing for personal income during your disability. Further, a good policy will not conflict with the payoff of an insurance policy providing for your disability. The cost for the overhead insurance is usually less than that for disability and is tax deductible. The benefits of this policy are taxable, but the premiums are charged off as business expenses. The policy covers all expenses except the cost of equipment, pharmaceuticals, and dentists' salaries. It does cover staff salaries.

Medical Insurance

Besides protecting the disability or the loss of income, you have to consider paying for any medical expenses through your medical insurance, which is composed of *basic health* and *major medical*. The basic health policy provides first-dollar coverage for inpatient/outpatient care and is very expensive. This should be supplemented by major medical, which picks up where the basic health leaves off.

For example, if your basic health was limited to $5,000, you would want a major medical policy to pick up expenses over $5,000. It is important to coordinate the upper and lower limits of your medical insurance policies.

Liability Insurance

When considering liability insurance, the first thought that comes to mind is malpractice insurance, the lack of which can lead to financial and professional disaster. The malpractice insurance should be purchased and in effect before you set foot into your new practice. The malpractice insurance must provide for claims which arise from failure to render, or rendering inadequate dental services. You should also be sure that there is no gap in coverage when changing policies. The factors to consider are that minimum coverage should equal $100,000 per claim, $300,000 aggregate per year, and you might consider at a very low cost the additional umbrella liability policy of $1 million, which will also cover auto liability and other non-professional liability. Specialists and general anesthesia users should certainly have $1 million coverage.

It is important when purchasing the liability policy to determine the basis for the coverage. Those policies which cover on an *occurrence basis* provide protection for treatment rendered regardless of the year in which the claim is filed. On the other hand, a *claims made* policy will provide coverage only while the insurance is in effect. In other words, if you are accused of malpractice after you retire from your practice, the occurrence basis coverage would protect you from the malpractice suit. However, in the claims made case, if you had dropped your insurance after retiring from your practice, you would not have protection from the malpractice claim.

It is also important to determine who is covered, keeping in mind that you are responsible for negligent acts of your staff, particularly to make sure that if you are in an associateship, that the associate is also covered. Further, liability insurance will not protect the assistants or hygienists if they are sued separately. If you are in a corporation, the corporation as well as the members should be covered. Also, partners may be held responsible for each other's malpractice acts.

It is also important to decide what is covered. Criminal acts (torts) are not covered under any malpractice policy. Malpractice policies will cover defense costs and judgments and should insure that you have the final right to make the decision as to whether to settle in or out of court. Be sure to check that the policy insures against all dental procedures that you intend to utilize.

Premises insurance is a form of liability insurance which protects for injuries incurred on the premises plus protection against water and fire damage. You must be sure that you are insured for at least 80 percent of the total value of the property. If not, only the depreciated cost of any damage will be paid. If you have covered 80 percent of the value, then the replacement cost is provided.

Normally, insurance companies will give you the option of purchasing a policy which automatically increases the coverage based upon inflation. This will help to guard against the possibility of coverage dropping below 80 percent, but even this does not provide assurance of adequate coverage. You should have periodic appraisals to establish the value of your facility, especially when market values are fluctuating widely.

A liability coverage which is frequently overlooked is that of a *non-owned auto coverage,* which will cover you if one of your staff has an accident while driving her own car to conduct business for the practice.

You should also consider coverage for the operatory, office equipment, in-transit loss, office records (accounts receivable) and money which are not covered by normal fire coverage. The *accounts receivable insurance* covers loss against uncollectable accounts receivable due to the loss of records. Additionally, you need to take a look at *practice-interruption insurance,* which covers the costs of setting up new or temporary offices in the event of damage to the original premises.

Next, we will cover some considerations in the purchase of insurance. One is the tax consideration. Normally, professional liability and coverage for office property are deductible as costs of doing business. However, in each case, you should check carefully with your CPA.

Whether to purchase from one or several companies is another frequently asked question. It is generally better to purchase from one company, since one policy and one billing procedure should prevent the possibility of a lapse in the policy. It also prevents disallowance for overlapping coverages wherein one company will not pay because similar coverage is held in another company, therefore causing you to lose the payments from both companies. It is also important to be sure that the policy clearly defines the differences between office premise liability and professional liability.

For example, if a patient falls getting out of the chair, it could be classified under either policy and may, if it were carried by more than one company, not be covered under either policy. Generally, dealing with one company can also result in lower rates. It is also important to purchase your insurance from reputable companies supported by the ADA whose professional protection plan is available in all states except California.

Now let's talk about organizing your insurance program. First it is important to examine and recognize ways you can suffer loss. Organize your program so that you are sure that all of the risks that you desire to have covered are covered. Then follow the guides for buying insurance economically by buying to insure risk and not by trying to use the insurance policy as an investment program. Get professional advice as to the coverage of, and the tax implications for, each policy. Then carefully study the insurance costs. A good way to compare insurance costs is to compare cost per $1,000 of coverage per year, which highlights the differences in costs of the policies. Decide what risks to insure against and how much loss you might suffer in each. For example, it would be ridiculous to purchase $1 million worth of insurance against a risk which has one chance in five billion of ever occurring, such as your being struck by lightning while in the basement of an apartment building.

Once you decide what risks you wish to insure against, cover your largest exposure first, using as high a deductible as you can afford. The use of deductible insurance is very handy, since it protects you against catastrophe while greatly reducing the premiums. Be sure to avoid duplication, use package units where possible, and periodically review your policies as your situation changes.

Summary

Insurance programs are provided by companies who are willing to assume or share portions of the risks you face such as death, disability, damage suits, etc. Of course, companies must charge you for the amount of risk they share, so you must carefully evaluate the degree of risk you face to determine how much you wish the insurance companies to assume. It is wasteful to pay high prices for a small amount of risk that you can take yourself. The deductible provisions of the insurance policies allow you to make this determination. Keep in mind that insurance is part of a risk management, not an investment program. Shop carefully for your insurance and read the policies thoroughly to make sure you are getting the coverage you desire.

Review Questions

1. Why should all liability insurance be purchased from one company?
2. If you receive life insurance paid for by a corporation, what portion of the premiums or settlement do you or your heirs pay taxes on?
3. In general, what type of life insurance policies provide the most protection for the least amount of money?

17
Computers in a Dental Practice

Learning Objectives

Upon completion of this chapter, you should be able to:

- Describe the basic components of the computer system and how these components function in support of dental practice management.
- Develop the criteria for a dental practice management software package.

Introduction

The purpose of this chapter is to familiarize you with the use of computers in a dental practice. Because so much has been written on computers in small businesses, including the dental practice, only an overview of the subject will be covered here.

There are several reasons why dentists want to computerize their practices:

- to streamline their operation
- to provide more information on which to base decisions
- to provide better service to the patient
- to organize an unorganized practice

Computerization will not cure a disorganized practice; it may even make conditions worse. To use a computer effectively requires a very structured and disciplined practice, because the computer must receive its information in a very exact way. It cannot discern good information from bad information.

Computer System Options

Once you have decided to computerize your practice, the next step is to decide the best way to go about it. You have three options:

1. to employ a service bureau
2. to share a computer
3. to have your own in-house computer

Service bureaus maintain large computers and provide packaged services to meet your requirements. The simplest service is to provide automatic billing in which you provide the service bureau with basic information through the mail, such as copies of your patient ledger cards from which the bureau generates your billings.

From this simple arrangement, services can be expanded to provide aging of accounts receivable, maintaining payroll records and other disbursement records, and providing balance sheets and income statements.

The service bureau may furnish this service by what is known as *batch processing*, or *real-time processing*. The batch processing method accumulates your input data and produces the output in a batch at a specific time or time interval such as the monthly billings. The shortcoming of this system is that you have no access to the information in the meantime and must rely on your own manual system to provide information on patient accounts and other requirements.

Real-time processing permits you to enter and retrieve data from the bureau's computer through the use of a remote terminal in your office. The amount of information available is negotiable and can vary from a limited amount of information such as the status of a patient's bill to the full data provided by the bureau.

In choosing between these two alternatives, you must consider the cost, with the real-time system being the more expensive. (However, the cost is not as large as you might think, for the major cost to the service bureau is the cost of the personnel used to feed your information into the computer.) Your other major consideration is to insure that the system provides you with a reasonable means of detecting and correcting errors and provides a reasonable turnaround or response time. Some data will not require a rapid turnaround time, such as accounts receivable aging, while one- to two-minute turnaround time is unacceptable when answering a telephone query about the patient's balance, or when trying to schedule a patient.

The next step up in attaining a computer capability is the purchase or rental of an in-house computer. Since the microcomputer has sufficient capacity for the average dental practice, we will limit our discussion to these small computers. Despite the fact that they are small, they are not inexpensive. The microcomputer used in our clinic is available for approximately $11,000, depending on the negotiations with the vendor. This price includes the software, printer, and hard disk memory.

Microcomputer Components

The typical microcomputer used in a dental practice consists of an input device which looks like a typewriter keyboard. Inside this keyboard are computer chips, some of which are permanently installed and others which are mounted on small cards which can be quickly and easily removed or installed. These chips provide the memory storage and operating programs for the microcomputer system. For example, additional chips can be installed to further increase the computer's memory capacity.

The operating programs themselves take up a portion of the available memory. They direct the operation of the computer system by issuing instructions to read input from input devices, process the input data as directed, store and retrieve data from memory during the processing, and display the output either in printed form or on the monitor.

The input and output data may be stored for future use in three ways. The simplest way is to use a cassette tape recorder, which has entry and retrieval times that are too slow to be of practical use in a dental office. The practical storage systems are the floppy diskettes and the hard disk.

The floppy diskettes are 3½", 5¼", or 8" flexible disks on which the data is electronically stored.

A 5¼" disk has a capacity of approximately 25,000 words. A disk drive is required in order to enter and retrieve data from the disks. These drives are either built into the input device or connected to the input device through a cable and what is known as an interface card. Four 5" drives are normally sufficient to operate a dental program in an office with up to 1,550 patients, while a dual 8" drive will handle up to 2,000 patients.

The other alternative is the use of a hard disk which operates in a manner very similar to the floppy disk drives. However, it has a much greater storage capacity, and because disks do not have to be inserted and removed from the drive, it is much faster in operation. Normally, hard disks are labeled by their size in megabytes. A 20 megabyte hard disk can store as much data as 115 diskettes. There is a drawback to some hard disks in that they are annoyingly noisy, so arrangements must be made to shield the disk drive from the staff.

No business computer system can be complete without a hard copy output device such as a printer to provide for billing schedules and other important practice data. There are two main types of printers: the *daisy wheel*, which prints a *letter-quality* output, and the *dot matrix printer*, which is considered by many to be inferior in appearance to the daisy wheel. However, the dot matrix printer is less expensive, faster, and far more versatile than the daisy wheel since it can be used for graphics and can easily be programmed to print in different sizes. If there are a sufficient number of dots in the print head — for example, a 9 × 9 matrix — the appearance is very close to the quality of the daisy wheel.

If you do not need the full capacity of the hard disk, switching systems and communications devices are available at reasonable prices which will permit you to share your computer with other dentists by transmitting data over wire or telephone lines between offices. The system also provides a series of security devices to insure that those sharing computers can only access their own data.

Determining Computer Requirements

Once you have decided to investigate how a computer may improve your practice, there are a number of steps that may be taken to insure that you make the right decision and, if that decision is to computerize, that the implementation will go smoothly. The first step is the same as the one we discussed in Chapter 1: *Plan!* You must once again review your practice objectives and the activities required to meet those objectives. If the objectives and activities are still sound, ask yourself how the computer will help you accomplish those activities.

To take some examples, suppose the following were one of your practice objectives: "To reduce the accounts receivable collection time to less than 60 days."

You must now outline exactly how the computer will be used to support these activities. For example:

1. The system will provide for inputting the patient's charge at point of departure from the office. A means must also exist to indicate whether or not the patient paid and to compute the unpaid balance, which must be printed immediately in bill form for presentation to the patient along with a statement of the practice credit policy.
2. The computer must issue a printed statement every 30 days, indicating the balance due for individual patients plus computing and adding the interest charge on all balances due over 30 days.
3. At the end of each month, the computer must age all accounts receivable and provide a written report indicating the percent of gross tied up in each of the following categories: 30, 60, 90, and 180 days.
4. Print a list of patients to whom the 180-day warning is to be sent, and after approval, print the individual warnings along with the mailing labels for mailing.

This procedure provides you with a list of functions which the computer must accomplish to support this one objective. You must repeat the procedure for each of your practice objectives. The end result will provide you with the *documentation* or criteria which the computer system must meet to fulfill all your objectives. Before you start the search for a computer system, you should prioritize the functions so that you can make decisions as to how much you are willing to pay for each additional function.

In prioritizing your requirements, you might want to think of three major areas in which the computer can be used. These are (1) billing and accounting, (2) patient dental records, and (3) patient scheduling. In the past, most dentists assigned their number one priority to the billing and accounting function and had not placed much emphasis on the other two functions. I would place patient scheduling second in priority, with special emphasis on tracking and scheduling the recall patient. Experience has shown that it takes approximately three months to complete one month's recall patients. This entails first the determination of what patients are due for recall in a given month, then sending the recall notice to those patients.

Then two follow-up notices spaced thirty days apart should be sent to those patients who do not respond.

Computer programs can be of immeasurable assistance in streamlining these procedures. The computerization of dental records would take a last priority unless the practice has grown to the point that space for normal dental records is not available. As an example of the need for prioritizing, one software company provides the basic functions plus appointment scheduling, telephone insurance filing, and treatment plan as separate modules at an additional price of $300 each.

Once you have decided on the functions you want your computer system to perform, you have a set of criteria against which to evaluate available software packages. Notice that we have not mentioned hardware at all to this point. The software is the important part of the system. Once you have determined the software package that will meet your criteria, you can then find the proper hardware to operate the software.

Procuring a Computer

It is normally best to seek the *vertical markets* when searching for your computer system. Vertical markets are vendors who deal in software for specialized fields such as dentistry, medical, or financial. These vendors will not only be able to provide the software, but will also be able to recommend the proper hardware and firmware to round out the system.

In narrowing your search, look for large companies who have been in business for several years. The computer market is very volatile, and companies come and go at a rapid rate, as evidenced by the recent bankruptcy of the Osborne computer company. You want to be sure that the company will remain in existence for the life of your computer system.

The other recommendation is to seek out present users of the system for their comments and recommendations. I would place little faith in the recommendations of someone who has used the system less than a year. Normally, within a year all the functions of the system will have been exercised at least once. That is, all the financial functions will have had one complete cycle. For example, after running a system for 9 months, I would have recommended it; however, in the tenth month we added an associate to the practice and entered the data into the computer, only to find that the system would not permit the changing of the number of the dentists except at the end of a year! The only way the system could be operated was to zero all accounts and start over again. Obviously, after this experience, I would not recommend that system to anyone until such shortcomings were corrected.

Once you have decided on the system, you must carefully plan the implementation phase. This will consist of delivery and installation of the system, loading the computer with all the practice data, training your staff, and running the system in parallel with the previous management system until you are certain that the system is reliable before dropping the old system.

Unless you are very lucky, the implementation phase will take at least twice as long as estimated. I would strongly recommend that you contract not only for the training, but for the loading of the practice data into the computer. To try to load the data into the computer while your staff are still inexperienced in the operation of the system will normally result in the introduction of numerous errors, which will cause frustration and lengthy delays in attaining an operational system.

One last caution: Be sure that you have a reliable backup system and that the system is backed up daily, for sooner or later the system will fail and only a reliable backup system properly implemented will save you from disaster.

Summary

American Dental Association study groups found that computers could increase the efficiency of a dental practice and predicted a larger role for computers in dentistry. The computer can provide more information organized in a manner which will facilitate your decision making. When determining the need for a computer, you must carefully analyze the objectives of your practice and then specifically define exactly how the computer can help you achieve those objectives. The end result should be a list of criteria for selecting the software required for your practice. Choose the software first, and buy from an established company with a reliable reputation.

Review Questions

1. Discuss the pros and cons of three computer options available to your dental practice.
2. Set up the goals of your recall system and define exactly how a computer could assist you in meeting your goals.

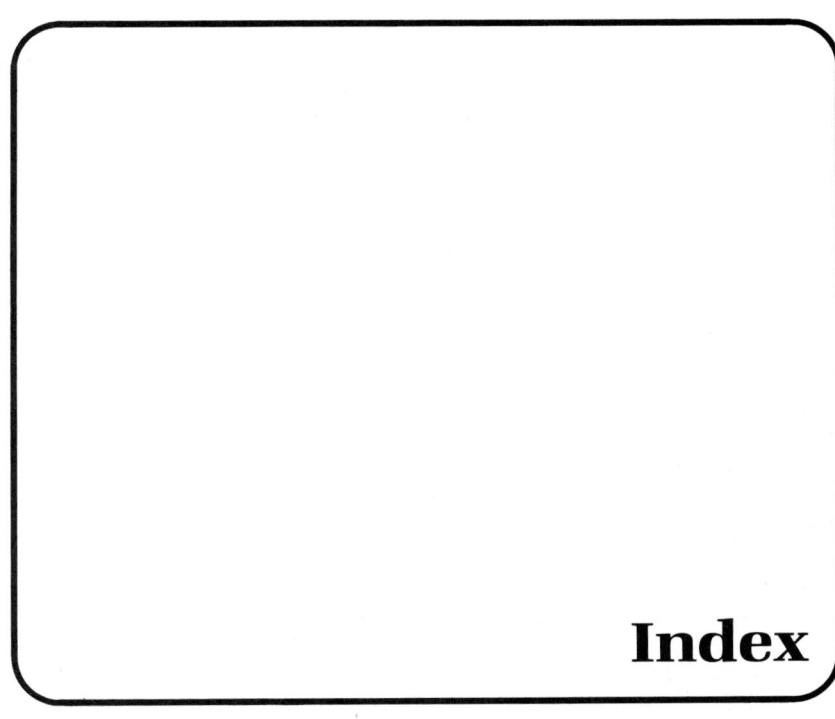

Index

Absenteeism, 73
Accounting, accrual, cash, 164
Accounting system
  Billing, 143
  Disbursement, 143
  Pegboard, 140
Accounts receivable, 147
  Aging, 37
  Collection rate, 37
Advertising, 120, 125
Agenda, staff meeting, 65
Analysis, non-financial, 182
Appointment plan, time units, 132
Assets, 163
Associateship, agreement, 45

Balance sheet, 163
Behavior—task relevant, 54, 65

Biases
  Hiring, 89
  Performance appraisal, 113
Bona fide occupational qualification, 85
Breakeven formula, 38, 179
Breakeven point, 177
Buy-sell agreement, 47, 195

Closed panel, 150
Cohesiveness, 73
Collection agencies, 149
Compensation, associateship, 38
Conflict
  Indicators, 78
  Staff meetings, 69
  Win-lose, 68
Contingency theory, 51
Contribution to margin, 179, 191

Costs
   Fixed, 40
   Variable, 40
Credit bureau, 148

Day sheet, 140
Decision making
   Considerations, 98
   Model, 101
   Participation, 103
   Staff development, 103
Delta plan, 150
Demand deposits, 19
Dentist-to-population ratio, 19
Dentist utilization, 188
Depreciation, 164
Discrimination, 83
Disk, hard, 206
Diskette, 206

Economic factors, and practice location, 18
Escape clause, 23
Evaluating a practice, 25
Expenses
   Fixed, 177
   Variable, 177

Feedback, 65
Fees, usual, customary, reasonable, 152
Forecasting, 7

Goal setting
   Management by objectives, 11
   Participation, 10
      Feedback, 11
      Rewards, 11
Goals, performance, 115
Goodwill, 31, 37
Group
   Cohesiveness, 73
   Norms, 73, 75

Hierarchy of effects, 124

Income statement, 169
Income statement, comparative, 171
Independent contractor, 43
Insurance
   Guaranteed renewable, 195
   Noncancellable, 197
Interviews—hiring, 87

Job
   Description, 80
   Specifications, 81

Key result areas, 13

Leader behavior, 51
Leadership
   Contingency theory, 51
   Effective vs. successful, 53
Leasing, 23
Ledger
   Card, 140
   Daily, 140

Malpractice, 199
Management by objectives, 12
Manager skills, 49
Marketing
   Definition, 120
   Plan, 120
   Segmentation, 121
   The four Ps, 121
Markets, vertical, 208
Maturity, follower, 55
Motivation, paradigm, 111

Net income, desired, 40
Norms, 75

Objectives
   Business, 5
   Criteria, 6
   Innovative, 6
   Problem solving, 14
Office manual, 63
Overhead, 177

Pareto principle, 13
Participation
  Decision making, 103
  Goal setting, 10
Patient contact time, 188
Patient management
  Appointment plan, 131
  Overhead time, 131
  Prime time, 131
  Waiting time, 130
Performance control, 10
Performance standards, 13, 115
Planning
  Action steps, 9
  Definition, 1
  Forecasting, 7
  Goal attainment, 13
  Goals, 4
  Process, 3
Practice location
  Demographic factors, 19
  Personal factors, 18
  Professional factors, 20
Pricing the practice, 28
Processing
  Batch, 204
  Real time, 204

Proof of posting, 140
Purpose
  Life, 3
  Practice, 3

Ratio
  A/R to gross income, 174
  Capital turnover, 173
  Current, 173
  Return on investment, 174
  Variable expense, 177
Recruiting, steps, 87
Restrictive covenant, 29
Risk management, 194

Selection checklist, 83
Skills, of a manager, 49
Staff meeting
  Agenda, 65, 67
  Stand up, 64, 70

Taxes, and independent contractor, 43
Team building, 65
Third-party payments, 150

Variable expense, 177
Variable expense ratio, 177